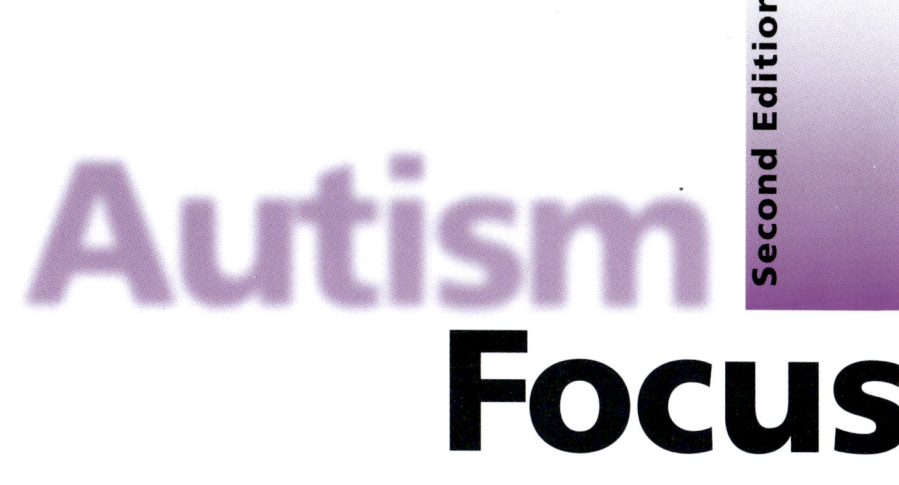

Autism
Second Edition

Focus

THE TRAINING WORKBOOK FOR PROFESSIONALS

CW01561640

Written by
Tom McKernan
and John Mortlock

CONTENTS

FOREWORD

There are, as yet, no known methods of curing autistic disorders. There are no known ways of repairing or even modifying the impairments of brain development that underlie the disabilities and behavioural features of this group of conditions. Many claims have been made about so-called treatments that range from the superficially plausible to the totally bizarre, but there is no independent evidence that any of them work.

This does not mean that nothing can be done. Special educational methods enable the children to develop any skills they may have to their fullest potential so that they can be used in adult life for pleasure and profit. However, whatever their ages, people with autistic disorders are deeply affected by the environment and daily programme in their home and work place. For adults in day or residential care and sheltered work, these environments are created by the care staff and work supervisors. The design of the buildings has an influence, for good or ill, but it is the human beings who have the real responsibility for the happiness and wellbeing of those for whom they care. But living and working with people with autistic disorders is not like living and working with anyone else with or without disabilities. Past experience of social interaction and a desire to help are not sufficient guides. It is essential to understand the nature of autistic conditions. People with these disorders, because of their social impairments, cannot meet you half-way. You have to make an imaginative leap into their world and try to see things from their point of view. This cannot be achieved by using ordinary social instincts because autism presents too many unexpected facets and paradoxes of behaviour. Parents learn the hard way by living with their children. Staff coming new to the work need special training to help them make sense of the autistic world.

In 1995 Tom McKernan and John Mortlock produced the first manual for training staff working with adults with autistic disorders. This has subsequently been revised and updated in a second edition. Their approach is clear, practical and systematic. They address the triad of impairments of social interaction, communication and imagination, and the repetitive pattern of activities that are the core problems present in all forms of autistic disorders. They give clear examples of autistic behaviour, discuss ways of helping, and set out exercises for those in training that are well designed to stimulate thought and increase understanding of the nature of autism.

The authors have undertaken a difficult task and have succeeded admirably in their aims. This manual should be used for basic training of staff in all residential and day centres where adults with autism live or work.

Lorna Wing
Consultant Psychiatrist, Centre for Social and Communication Disorders
Founder member, Sussex Autistic Society

Autism Focus is a course of training for workers who care for people with autistic spectrum disorders. It converts theory into care practice, enabling the skills and competence of care professionals to be developed, and concentrates on those areas which make the care of people with autism different from other groups of people.

This workbook takes a step-by-step approach, guiding you through your study and providing you with all the information you need. However, it is best that you have a study supervisor who can help you when you need clarification and support. It may also be helpful to have some background reading material available, and a suggested list is given on page iii.

The workbook includes an introductory level of specialist training which should be completed before starting the rest of the material. The course will help you to look at some of the behaviours and special needs of people with autism in depth and devise care plans which will help them to overcome their difficulties.

In Section 1 you are asked to identify clients whose behaviours appear to match those described as examples of the behaviours often seen amongst people with autism. You will quickly realise that you are unlikely ever to see all these behaviours in one person, but you will see most of them amongst any group of people who have the impairments of autism.

The *Autism Focus* workbook has been divided into four sections, each containing a number of worksheets to be completed. The course has been designed to stretch you, as well as deepen your understanding of how to respond to the special needs of people with autism. Before you start work on it, spend some time with the person who is to be your study supervisor. Look through the material and discuss any problems you can foresee.

Take your time working through this programme; there are no prizes for speed and trying to complete it in the minimum time possible is likely to mean missing out on important observations and learning. Some of the worksheets ask you to carry out observations over a week, and there are a lot of worksheets. Setting yourself the goal of completing *Autism Focus* over a six-month period is fast enough.

Value your workbook and look after it, for it will provide a useful source of information and ideas for years to come. Complete the worksheets only when you are entirely happy with your work. Until then, keep a loose-leaf folder with your notes and 'rough work'. You will also find space in the workbook to make notes and clarifications for future reference.

Further reading you may find useful

The Autistic Spectrum – book – by Lorna Wing. Published by Constable 1996.

The Handbook of Autism – book – by Aarons and Gittens. Published by Routledge, second edition 1999.

Autism: The Facts – book – by Simon Baron-Cohen and Patrick Bolton. Published by the Oxford University Press 1993.

Nobody Nowhere – book – by Donna Williams. Published by Doubleday 1992.

Thinking in Pictures – book – by Temple Grandin. Published by Vintage Books 1996

Asperger Syndrome – book – by Tony Attwood. Published by Jessica Kingsley 1998

Autism and Asperger Syndrome – book – edited by Uta Frith. Published by Cambridge University Press 1991.

COMPLETING THE WORKBOOK

As you work through this training programme you will learn to approach the care and training of people with autistic spectrum disorders in a more analytical and structured way. You will practise observing, interpreting and recording behaviours. You will practise devising interventions which overcome some of the difficulties people with autism experience.

Notes

The Exercises

These are intended to make you think about the particular issue you are working on at the time. You will be asked to make observations, both of your own behaviour and that of the clients, and then discuss these with your study supervisor.

You will notice that you have experienced some of the problems your clients have to face, but not as acutely. None of the feelings experienced by the clients are different from your own, though they may find them harder to cope with. Very few of the behaviours which are displayed by clients are peculiar to people with autism. Only the degree to which they are presented, the places where they occur, or their frequency, are different.

Make notes as directed in the space provided or, if you prefer, on a separate sheet, and discuss these with your study supervisor. You may not wish to discuss every detail which is personal to you but you will be expected to share your findings.

The Worksheets

In all the sections you will find worksheets which you will need to complete. Depending on your personal needs or those of the organisation you work for, most, if not all, may have to be completed as evidence of the learning you have achieved. If you are doing an NVQ in Care, a completed workbook will provide evidence of your ability to respond to the specialised individual needs of your clients. However, as a general guide it should not be necessary to complete absolutely every worksheet to provide evidence. Guidelines on the satisfactory level of evidence is given below.

The worksheets provide evidence of your ability to observe and analyse behaviours which result from autism, and to devise effective ways of responding to them. Some worksheets offer the opportunity to demonstrate your insights into the condition. It may be that they prompt you to consider ways of working with clients which differ from the way you work now. In this case DO NOT attempt to change your way of working with that person until you have discussed your ideas with your supervisor and line manager.

Notes
....

If you have difficulty in identifying a suitable client in your unit for a particular exercise or task, speak to your line manager who may be able to suggest somebody in another department or site.

It is suggested that, as a minimum, you complete the worksheets as detailed below:

INTRODUCTION

Complete all four worksheets.

COMMUNICATION

Complete the worksheet:

- communication.

WORKING WITH THE TRIAD

Impairment of social interaction

Choose four topics and complete the worksheets, from:

- isolated
- no eye contact
- joins in only if others insist
- bizarre behaviour and mannerisms
- inappropriate laughing or giggling
- displays indifference
- approaches people inappropriately.

Impairment of social communication

Choose two topics and complete the worksheets, from:

- echolalia
- one-sided interaction
- talks and thinks incessantly about one topic
- inappropriate display of emotions.

Impairment of imagination and social understanding

Choose one topic and complete the worksheet, from:

- change is not welcome
- uses objects without awareness of their use

- unaware of common dangers
- must have things exactly in place.

REPETITIVE BEHAVIOURS

Complete all three worksheets:

- observation of repetitive behaviour
- positive rituals
- overcoming problem behaviour.

CONSISTENT WORK PRACTICES

Complete the worksheet:

- consistent work practice.

Please be sure to remember when completing the worksheets that you are observing and analysing behaviour and not personality. It is important not to label someone with a 'personality type' on the basis of their behaviour.

Remember that behaviour can be changed whereas a label, once securely attached, is often very difficult to remove.

As well as the worksheets, your study supervisor will require evidence that you have properly completed the exercises, and gained learning and insight in the process.

Do not worry if there are not enough people with autism in the place where you work for you to be able to complete all the worksheets. For now it is enough to address some of the problems which those in your care may be experiencing. It may be that you will have the opportunity to work with more people with autism in the future. You will then be able to return to your workbook for ideas and guidance, and then be able to complete more worksheets.

STUDY SUPERVISOR'S GUIDANCE

As a senior staff member or line manager, you may be called upon to act as a study supervisor. You may feel that you do not have the expertise in autism to fulfil this role, or you may lack the confidence to supervise someone's study.

Notes

Notes

Do not worry. Being a study supervisor is not a matter of showing off your knowledge, nor of setting yourself up as an expert. Your role is to ensure that the person you are supervising learns new knowledge and skills, and in the process, gain more expertise yourself. Be prepared to learn with the person you are supervising – by learning together you will share an enriching experience and will probably find that learning is more enjoyable.

Meet regularly to review the progress that the person you are supervising is making. Remember to check not only the worksheets but also for evidence of learning from the exercises.

LEARNING CIRCLES

If you are unable to find a study supervisor, an alternative to solitary learning is to get together with another person, or even form a group. It would be helpful if you all worked in the same unit but it is not essential. If you are the only person studying *Autism Focus* where you work, try looking elsewhere or advertising for study partners on a notice board, newsletter or other means.

By combining your knowledge, efforts and experience you will discover the truth in the old saying that two heads are better than one. A learning circle can be a great support, and encouragement, progress and success are much more likely in the company of others who share similar aims.

The authors would like to receive your comments about the Autism Focus training programme, and any suggestions you may have for improving it. Please address your comments and suggestions to:

Sussex Autistic Community Trust
Unit 5, Ore Business Park
Hastings
East Sussex
TN35 5QA

Telephone: 01424 715955
Fax: 01424 715956

WHAT IS AUTISM?

Autism is a disorder of development which affects at least 120,000 people in Great Britain. Some 75% of these people also have a degree of learning disability, ranging from mild to very severe. The majority of these people need some form of support service to help them survive in society and, hopefully, gain some independence to help them to live as normally as possible.

The words 'autistic' and 'autism' come from the Greek word 'autos' which means 'self'. The reason this word is used to describe this group of people relates to their isolation from normal social behaviour.

Autism affects more males than females; a ratio of approximately 4:1 overall. However, with severe or profound learning disabilities, the excess of males is much less marked. It affects people with all levels of intellectual ability, varying from profound learning disability to average or superior ability. Autism affects people of all classes, races and creeds.

You may have already noticed that people with autism do not necessarily fall into a convenient stereotype but can appear to be very different from each other. There are a number of reasons for this:

- Autism is caused by the combination of three particular impairments, each of which can vary in severity.

- In addition to these three impairments, people with autism can be affected by learning disability, which can also vary in severity.

- Each person with autism has their own individual personality and is a unique individual, just as you are.

Asperger syndrome

Asperger syndrome is sometimes referred to as high functioning autism or mild autism. It is generally agreed that people with this syndrome are part of the autism spectrum. Such individuals are better able to communicate by virtue of their language abilities, but still suffer from the social communication problems and social ineptness of all people with autistic disorders.

People with Asperger syndrome are usually noticeable by their odd and circumscribed interests. These interests will often form their sole topic of conversation and they will insist on talking about this subject regardless of whether the other person is interested or has heard it all before.

Notes

They will typically be of average or above average intelligence and their intense focus of interest will sometimes lead to remarkable achievements. Feats of memory and mathematical prowess are common but they inevitably have great difficulty in activities which require social skills or co-operation.

AUTISM – A DIAGNOSIS

During their study of the population of the London Borough of Camberwell in the 1970s, Drs Lorna Wing and Judy Gould studied the social behaviour of children, trying to identify those whose social behaviour was inappropriate to their mental age. They found that impairment of social relating skills was closely linked to two other areas of social impairment: impairment of social communication and impairment of imagination and social understanding.

In the study, this group of three impairments (the 'triad') was found in all the children who had typical autism, as first described by the psychiatrist, Leo Kanner, working in the USA in the 1940s. However, Wing and Gould also found many other children with the triad who did not have typical autism, but who had many of the features described by Kanner and who had exactly the same special needs as those who were typically autistic. Wing and Gould suggested that there was a spectrum (or continuum) of conditions that have the triad of impairments in common. These are not illnesses, but disorders of development of the social, communication and imagination skills that should normally emerge in infancy and early childhood.

Summary of essential features

The following clinical features are characteristic of people with autistic spectrum disorders

Wing's Triad of Impairments

1. Impairment of social interaction

2. Impairment of social communication

3. Impairment of imagination and social understanding

Repetitive behaviours

These include simple ones such as flicking fingers or objects, tapping, rocking, etc, and complex ones such as insistence on following routines, obsession with particular activities (eg train spotting, computers), obsession with collecting objects (especially those with no apparent intrinsic value), obsession with collecting facts (eg pop trivia, cars).

Notes

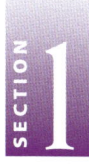

Examples of characteristics commonly found in people with autism:

- indifference to others
- aloofness
- one-sided in social interaction
- uses others mechanically
- play not creative or co-operative
- incessant single-topic talk
- display of emotion inappropriate to situation
- echolalic speech
- lack of eye contact
- manipulates objects regardless of their real use
- exceptionally skilled in a single activity
- intense resistance to change
- persistent problems with relationships.

UNDERSTANDING THE TRIAD OF IMPAIRMENTS

When carrying out assessments and planning care and training activities it is particularly important to consider the implications of a diagnosis of autism. It is the responsibility of care staff to develop a good understanding of the condition. Below are some explanations of how the triad affects their ability to relate to other people and to their environment.

The diagnosis of autism carries with it the expectation that there will be factors which should have an influence on care planning, different from those of other groups of people. These factors were identified by Wing as the Triad of Impairments, namely:

Impairment of social interaction
Impairment of social communication
Impairment of imagination and social understanding.

Some of the characteristics of the Triad of Impairments are described overleaf.

Notes

Notes

Impairment of social interaction

This impairment affects different people's ability to relate to others in different ways; there is no one autistic stereotype. Three typical types of social interaction are identified as:

- *Aloof:* in its most severe form, the affected person will appear indifferent to other people, especially their peers. Sometimes they will seem to regard others as objects, even to the point of moving them out of their way. Many will use others mechanically to meet their needs, ie using the hand of a carer to try to unlock a door. However, many will form simple attachments, especially to familiar carers.

- *Passive:* the affected person may passively accept social contact, might even show some pleasure in this, but does not make spontaneous approaches. Some will attend a wide range of activities without complaint but only take part when led. Such people tend to be solitary and often engage in repetitive behaviours, such as twiddling, tapping, rocking, etc.

- *Active but odd:* some will approach other people spontaneously but do so in an odd, repetitive way, pay no attention to the response of the people they approach and fail to consider their point of view. Typically such an individual will engage others in a one-sided conversation or ask repetitive questions whilst paying little or no attention to the answers.

Many people with autism display all three types of behaviour, depending on the circumstances.

Among the more able adults who have the ability to adapt somewhat, the impairment may have evolved into an inappropriately stilted and formal manner of interaction with family and friends as well as strangers.

In Section 3 you will find some examples of how impairment of social interaction affects people with autism. In these examples you will see this list:

Range of Impairment:
Aloof
Passive
Active but Odd

This is to help remind you of the range of behaviours associated with this particular impairment and which you may come across when working with with people with autism.

Impairment of social communication

Adding to their difficulties in taking part in social interaction with others, people with autistic spectrum disorders have difficulty in using and understanding both verbal and non-verbal communication. Again there is a range of impairment and everybody is affected differently. Some of the ways people with autism may be affected are described below.

- *Absence of any desire to communicate with others:* describes those who do not readily use speech, signing or writing to communicate with others. Such people often have some understanding of words spoken by other people, though not always.

- *Echolalic and repetitive speech:* echolalia describes the way some people will respond to spoken language by repeating the words they have heard, rather than replying to them appropriately.

- *Communication confined to the expression of needs only:* describes those who have little interest in using their language skills until the events going on around them affect them directly. Speech or signing is only used to frame short statements, or to ask for things that the person wants.

- *Makes factual comments, often irrelevant to the situation:* this often occurs because the individual does not know what information they should provide in answer to a question or a situation.

- *Talks incessantly, regardless of the response by others:* these people want to make social contact with others, but fail to appreciate the need to allow a gap for the other person to talk if they want to, or to take notice of what others may be trying to say.

- *Displays distortions of the rules of language:* some people with autism have a wide vocabulary but sound odd when they speak because of difficulty in understanding the 'rules' of speech. Some have distinct problems, such as failure to reverse personal pronouns, eg: Question "Do you want a cup of tea?" Answer "Yes, you do want a cup of tea".

The overall difficulties in communication suffered by many people with autism means that they tend to be very literal people who are likely either to assume that words mean just what they say or who become confused by what we actually mean when we say things like: "John cried his eyes out." (Think about the literal meaning of this expression.)

Notes
....

Impairment of imagination and social understanding

This third element of Wing's Triad of Impairment in autism is perhaps the hardest to understand. It is referred to as an impairment of imagination because in children it is shown by the absence or abnormality of imaginative, pretend play. In adults the problem is shown by inflexibility of attitude, the inability to imagine consequences of actions and severe difficulty in imagining how other people think and feel.

Having this impairment does not mean that people with autism cannot take part in any activities that seem to need imagination. Some are good at art and some can take part in drama, including role playing. However, the art is often on one repeated theme and the dramatic roles have to be learned precisely rather than understood from the inside. Despite these limitations, such activities can be very helpful for people with autistic disorders.

Wing has described the range of impairment of imagination and social understanding as:

- *Difficulty understanding that others may have a different point of view:* research shows that the majority of people with autism have difficulty in understanding that the ideas or beliefs of another person may be different to their own. This inability makes it hard for them to judge (to imagine) what other people may be thinking and may be about to do next, which may help to explain why they find social interaction difficult.

- *Difficulty in imagining the future:* living as they have to without understanding of other people or their lives, people with autism have little or no concept that other things are going on elsewhere. They live in an immediate world of the here and now. They do not enjoy the rich inner world of thoughts and feelings about their environment, society, friends, peers and events which most of us take for granted and which provides us with reassurance and anticipation. They are not able to appreciate that other people act independently of them, influencing events, out of their sight. In consequence, they are not able to anticipate how others might react, what might happen next, how things might turn out. Unless they are specifically told what is going to happen next, what, why, where, when, and when it will end, they are likely to be fearful of the future and what it holds for them. Even the next few minutes will seem like a fearful eternity if you cannot anticipate what is going to happen next.

- *Difficulty in planning ahead:* without the ability to anticipate future events, they have great difficulty in organising themselves, even for the next few minutes. This results in a dependence on routine and on events happening in a consistent, predictable order, with no deviations. There is also a tendency towards insistence on achieving short-term objectives, such as that next cup of tea, which must be achieved before they can move on to anything else. Any change to their routine or expectations means that they revert to fearing what might happen next.

People with autism are likely to defend routine and sameness rigorously – their sense of security depends on it.

- *Inflexibility in applying written and unwritten social rules:* the society we live in is governed by complex social rules, some of which are written down (laws) and others which are generally understood (customs). People with autism often fail to understand these rules. Where they do understand them they often have difficulty in judging when it is socially acceptable to bend or break those rules. For example: school rules may say that pupils should be quiet and well-behaved in the school buildings at all times, yet the school may hold a disco one night, where pupils are expected to be loud and excitable.

- *Repetitive enacting of role, often copied without understanding:* some people with autism learn by copying what they see other people doing, or by doing what other people have told them to do. This does not mean that they will have understood why and when this particular thing should be done.

- *Difficulty in generalising concepts, inflexibility of thought:* many people with autism seem to have difficulty in understanding that what they learn in one situation can be applied to another similar situation. Learning to swim in one particular swimming pool does not mean that the person will necessarily understand that they can now swim in any swimming pool. Through inflexibility of thought individuals can believe that the colour, smell, size, shape, taste, etc of the pool they learnt to swim in are all part of swimming. Change any one of those factors and the person with autism may become insecure about their ability.

Inflexibility of thought is responsible for the way many people with autism tend only to understand the literal meaning of the words they hear. For example, when someone asks us to "wait a minute", we know that the person saying this really means that they will attend to us as soon as possible. The literal interpretation of this means something else… as *you* will know.

Notes

Notes
....

OTHER CONDITIONS ASSOCIATED WITH AUTISM

- *Repetitive behaviour*
  Autism is closely associated with repetitive behaviour, where the individual repeatedly carries out a set series of actions which have no apparent purpose or relationship to what is going on around them.

- *Obsessional interests*
  Autism is also associated with obsessional interests, where the individual keeps returning to one narrow area of interest, ignoring other activities around them. This intense focus on one subject can give rise to unusually high degrees of talent in that one narrow area, when compared to the individual's general level of learning.

- *Learning disability*
  Some 75% of people with autism have associated learning disabilities. Many of the 25% who have normal or above average levels of intelligence can manage without full-time specialist care services but can still need some help in managing their lives.

- *Epilepsy*
  A high proportion of people with autism also suffer from epilepsy, a disorder of brain function that can cause occasional loss of consciousness, with or without convulsions. It can also cause changes of behaviour over which the person has no control.

- *Heightened senses*
  Some people with autism appear to be hypersensitive to touch, or sound, or to bright light and strong colours, and smell. It remains uncertain if they feel, hear, see or smell things differently, or if they simply react more to the same level of sensory stimulation experienced by other people.

- *Behavioural problems*
  Behavioural problems, sometimes known as challenging behaviour, affect some, but certainly not all people with autism. They often appear to be caused by the high levels of stress and frustration suffered by people who have difficulty in relating and communicating with those around them.

The causes of autism

Nobody can yet be certain of the precise cause of autism but it is believed to be associated with brain damage, which in turn may be caused by a number of different factors, for example:

- physical trauma, such as during a difficult birth

- a number of genetic conditions, such as tuberous sclerosis

- a number of viral infections, before or after birth, such as rubella (German measles) during mother's pregnancy.

MANAGING PEOPLE WITH AUTISM

A diagnosis of autism does not mean that the person so described ceases to be an individual with their own particular needs, desires and idiosyncrasies.

As you will now be aware, the diagnosis covers a range of factors which include people with profound learning disability, as well as highly intelligent people who are profoundly disabled in the social sense.

The terms 'more able' and 'able autistic' or 'Asperger syndrome' are often used to describe certain people with good verbal, self-help or other skills. However all people with autism are equally disadvantaged in the social sense.

The particular features and characteristics you have been learning about are normal for people with autism and acceptance of these norms is an essential first step towards the provision of services.

For activity, training or management programmes to be successful, careful consideration of the common features and difficulties associated with autism needs to be given. These include:

- obsessions with one activity or thought process

- inflexible rituals which have to be completed before doing anything else

- resistance to changes in daily routines

- irrational fears of everyday objects

- temper tantrums which may appear to have no cause

- problems with sleeping

- problems with eating

- problems with toileting.

Notes

....

Notes

Where the special needs of people with autism are not understood, any of these, or any combination of them, can prove bewildering to staff who do not understand why these behaviours occur. An individual programme plan (IPP) system is required to help staff to manage these problems in a planned and structured way.

Communicating with people with autism

It is very important to realise that although a person with autism may have a good vocabulary and seems able to use language effectively, they may not have a proper understanding of the words they use. It is essential to remember that, whatever their apparent level of verbal ability, other visual means of communication must be considered such as: pictures, pictograms, pointing, demonstrating, makaton, etc.

Many people with autism respond very well to visual information such as: written timetables which they can keep; communication books with words, pictures or symbols which they can use as an aid to expressing themselves; activity sequence cards which contain key words, pictures or symbols to illustrate the series of actions which are required to complete an activity.

Many would go so far as to say that written or pictorial timetables for each individual person are essential to provide the structure and predictable environment which is so important for people with autism. However, these are only of benefit if staff ensure that the activities are actually carried out as planned.

Considering a living environment for people with autistic spectrum disorders:

Physical Environment
- Privacy and personal space are important but this must be balanced by adequate supervision of people who are often unaware of common dangers.
- Safety aspects of furniture and fittings are important.
- Robust furniture and fittings will reduce pressure on staff.
- Levels of physical security, both inside and out must be considered.
- Noise levels should be considered – hypersensitive hearing is common.
- Boundaries must be clearly defined.

Social Interaction
- Social interaction is usually stressful, sometimes even painful, for people with autism – staff behaviour and expectations must take account of this.

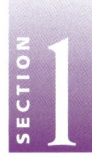

- They *do not* learn social behaviour merely from exposure to a sociable peer group.
- Their behaviour may well cause stress and anxiety to those with whom they live.
- Social mixing must be carefully planned to minimise distress.

Communication

- Social communication problems are normal for people with autism and to be expected, staff must learn to understand and communicate with each individual.
- Information should be presented in visual terms as much as possible.
- Staff should be aware of augmentative communication systems such as PECS, Makaton, Pic Symbols, etc. and be prepared to use them as appropriate.

Daily Programme

- **Must be structured and highly organised** with a timetable which is not subject to sudden, arbitrary changes and a staff rota which presents familiar staff in predictable patterns.
- Changes should always be planned in advance and carefully explained with reassurance. Sudden, arbitrary changes of plan should always be avoided.
- The timetable should be made readily available and presented pictorially for those who cannot read. A daily programme of activities in book form (pocket photo albums are useful) is also helpful, again presented pictorially if necessary.
- New activities should be introduced gradually and sensitively in small steps, by negotiation. Always have a contingency plan in case of refusal.
- A range of vigorous physical activities should be made available.
- An individual's skills and interests should be reflected in their programme.

Behaviour Management

- The atmosphere should at all times be calm and safe.
- The significance and importance of repetitive behaviours should be recognised, but effective strategies must be devised for limiting them and addressing the harmful ones. Such behaviours are often an indicator of anxiety, which must be addressed.
- Risk assessments must be carried out for all activities.
- Agreed and appropriate strategies must be devised for coping with disturbed or distressed behaviour.
- Psychologist support should be available to assist with devising strategies to cope with difficult behaviours.
- Psychiatric support may provide help with medication to reduce anxiety.

Notes

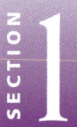

AUTISM – AN INTRODUCTION

Task 1

Name the features which are essential for a diagnosis of autism:

_____

_____

_____

_____

_____

_____

_____

_____

_____

_____

Task 2

Consider what you have learned in the section and use the information to select the correct word to complete the following statements:

Some people with autism are described as socially ALOOF because they appear to be…

1 aggressive   **2** friendly   **3** indifferent   **4** caring   …towards others.

Other people with autism are described as socially PASSIVE because they accept social contact when it is offered by others but do not make…

1 frequent   **2** spontaneous   **3** lasting   **4** physical   …contact themselves.

Some people with autism are socially ACTIVE and do make the first move in social interaction but their attempts to do this often appear ODD because they are often…

1 busy   **2** repetitive   **3** distracted   **4** preoccupied

…and do not pay attention to the…

1 appearance   **2** mood   **3** actions   **4** responses   …of other people.

WORKSHEET

2 | AUTISM – AN INTRODUCTION

Task 3

Difficulties with communication are about more than speech, they also include:

_____

_____

_____

_____

_____

_____

_____

_____

_____

_____

Task 4

Complete the following statement:

Impairment of imagination is about more than the ability to draw pictures or act out a role, it also affects:

_____

_____

_____

_____

_____

_____

_____

_____

_____

Notes

USING THE TRIAD OF IMPAIRMENTS TO UNDERSTAND INDIVIDUALS

The creation of individual programme plans (IPPs) depends on making accurate observations and recordings of the behaviour and skills of each individual you are caring for. In this programme you are learning to make observations of the particular behaviours associated with the Triad of Impairments.

Your next task is to select two clients and observe them over at least a week, using the information available in this section to identify the behaviours in terms of the Triad. Use worksheets 3 and 4, one for each client, to describe the behaviours which you can identify as indicating the impairments.

Discuss this project with your line manager and agree on the two clients you are going to observe over the period. The experience will be of greatest use to you if you choose two people who seem to be very different to each other. If you are not familiar with the process of making observations and recording them, ask for assistance.

You may end up with something like this example:

Impairment of social interaction
Joe is socially active but odd. He approaches staff holding out his hands, clearly wanting to relate to them. Once his hands are held he does not seem to know what to do next and turns away.

Impairment of social communication
Joe uses his communication skills to express his own needs only. He will not join in conversations but will repeatedly ask: "What's for tea?" and "Mum coming on Friday?", apparently taking no notice of the answers he is given.

Impairment of imagination and social understanding
Joe is inflexible in the application of rules. When he walks through the kitchen he will stop and put milk and butter back in the refrigerator when someone else is in the middle of using them.

He has difficulty in understanding that other people may have a different point of view as he seems to expect staff working with him in the evening to know what happened whilst he was at the day centre.

WORKSHEET
3

AUTISM – AN INTRODUCTION

TRIAD OF IMPAIRMENTS

Impairment of social interaction

Description of present behaviour
(You should have a particular client in mind, though it is not necessary to name him/her here)

_____

_____

_____

_____

_____

_____

Impairment of social communication

_____

_____

_____

_____

_____

_____

Impairment of imagination and social understanding

_____

_____

_____

_____

_____

_____

AUTISM – AN INTRODUCTION

TRIAD OF IMPAIRMENTS

Impairment of social interaction

Description of present behaviour
(You should have a particular client in mind, though it is not necessary to name him/her here)

_____

_____

_____

_____

_____

_____

Impairment of social communication

_____

_____

_____

_____

_____

_____

Impairment of imagination and social understanding

_____

_____

_____

_____

_____

_____

_____

UNDERSTANDING MEANING

You will realise by now that the difficulties that people with autistic spectrum disorders have with communication are not just in the expressive skills of speaking and writing. They also have difficulty understanding the meaning of what is communicated to them.

People with autistic spectrum disorders have difficulty understanding body language – the gestures and facial expressions we make whilst we speak. These gestures and facial expressions add meaning and emphasis to what we say, although we may be unaware of them in ourselves. Our body language also gives indications as to how we are feeling, clues for others which help them to respond appropriately.

People with autistic spectrum disorders have difficulty in understanding their environment and how things are connected. This means that they do not always recognise the links between the actions of others, how an action will have consequences, how several actions have to be organised in the correct order to achieve a desired outcome. They do not always understand the context in which activities and behaviours occur. In conversation, most of us take for granted our ability to 'fill in the gaps' as we converse; we do not always need everything explained in minute detail because we understand the links and the context, so can make do with a few clues and pointers.

Without the context, links, clues and pointers, people with autism are left with only the literal meaning of the words themselves. Consider the following exchange for example:

John (coming out of the office with a furious expression): "It's up the creek again!"

Sue (coming across John in the corridor): "It was only fixed yesterday! It's the third time this week, I'll have to get that clown back again – I'll haul him over the coals this time."

Sue *knows* that John is angry *because of the expression on his face*.
Sue *knows* that the cause of his anger is in the office *because of the context*.
Sue *knows* that there is no small stream involved *because of the context*.
Sue *knows* what it is that needs fixing *because she can link this incident with others*.
You *know* that Sue does not really get a clown to try and fix whatever it is.
You can *imagine* how frustrated they feel.

Notes

Notes

If just one word is added – you might choose from photocopier, printer, computer, etc – you can piece together the whole story. How can you do this?

We take this ability to fill in the gaps for granted, but what would we understand from the encounter without it? With only the literal meaning of the words we have an incomprehensible situation involving a small stream, a clown and some coals.

Without realising it, what we say is not always exactly what we mean. We have all sorts of ways of confusing the meaning of the things we say and of being inaccurate.

- We allude to things (drop hints or imply)
- We use colourful expressions ("don't get your knickers in a twist")
- We tell 'white lies' to spare the feelings of others ("yes, it looks lovely")
- We are ironic or even sarcastic ("oh that *was* a good idea, *wasn't it*?")
- We tell jokes (how many care workers does it take to change a light bulb?)

In spite of this we still understand what people mean and what is expected of us through the communication sub-texts of empathy, context, clues and pointers. People with autism, with only the literal meaning of the words to go on, have the greatest difficulty.

SEMANTIC PRAGMATIC DISORDER

You may have heard this term applied to people with autism, because it is common to them. Semantics and pragmatics are the ways in which words change their meaning because of context.

Semantics is the way in which the meaning of words is affected by the other words used with them. For instance the words *would* and *wood* sound the exactly the same and we only know which meaning to attach to the sound because of the accompanying words. So "I would like you to help me take the rubbish bins outside" has nothing to do with timber. However, people with autism might well take the sound of the word 'would' at the beginning of the sentence to mean timber and become stuck on thinking about different types of wood and thereby miss the request altogether.

Pragmatics is the way in which words change their meaning depending on what is happening around the speaker. So the question "Have you seen Fred?" would normally elicit more than a simple "yes" or "no" answer. Depending on what was happening at the time, it might be an opportunity to

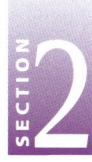

inform the questioner of Fred's whereabouts or the time of his arrival. Or alternatively it might be expected that you comment on his new hair cut.

People with autism have considerable difficulties with semantics and pragmatics. This leaves them to deal with the sounds of the words they hear in a literal way without reference to context or circumstance.

Consider how the following expressions can have unintended alternative meanings (in brackets) when spoken out loud:

I'd like to think of you and I	–	(I'd like to think of you and die)
Walk on ahead	–	(Walk on a head)
Go and see the new display	–	(Go and see the nudist play)
The window sill	–	(The window's ill)

Much of what we say is not intended to be taken literally. We use many expressions that are figurative. Consider how the following requests and suggestions should not be taken too literally:

See if you can catch the waiter's eye

Pop your head 'round the corner

Hop over to the counter

John needs a good kick up the backside

She died of embarrassment

UNDERSTANDING WHAT IS EXPECTED

It is not only semantics and pragmatics that cause problems with communication. Commonly, people with autism will give stock answers to questions that seem to answer them, but on closer inspection are not what they seem. Often they will seem to ignore a question or request, or give an answer might seem insolent. Consider some of the questions below and why they might be misunderstood.

Carer: "Would you like a beef burger or a hot-dog?"
David: "Hot-dog"
Carer: "Would you like a hot-dog or a beef burger".
David: "Beef burger".

David merely repeated the last thing he heard – he might not actually want either. He might not even realise that he has a choice.

Notes

Carer: "How are you today Sarala?"
Sarala: "Ivan wears yellow wellingtons" – giggles

Sarala always repeats those words when she is in a good mood. She has not seen Ivan (who wore funny yellow wellingtons) since she was at school, 10 years ago.

Carer: "How are you today Sarala?"
Sarala: "Tracy pulled my hair" – looks upset

Sarala always repeats those words when she is in a bad mood. She has not seen Tracy (who pulled her hair) since she was at school, 10 years ago.

Carer: "Will you clean up that mess please Adam"
Adam: "Hello"

Adam is not being awkward, he did not realise he was being spoken to until he heard his name, by which time the sentence was lost. He just responded to the sound of his name.

Carer: "Adam, will you clean up that mess please"
Adam: "No thank you"

If it was a request or instruction, why put it to Adam in the form of a question?

We often put requests and instructions to people in this way in order to be polite and not give the impression of being 'bossy'. Those of us on the receiving end of such a polite instruction tend to know that we are not being given a choice. Adam must be excused for assuming that he had been given a choice though because of his literal understanding of the words.

Carer: "Have you got a frog in your throat?"
Chris: "No!"

Well in point of fact she has not.

Cut adrift from the social context of their environment and without the ability to use language effectively as a tool for understanding others or expressing their feelings or needs, people with autism may be misunderstood and even blamed for being awkward and refusing to answer or comply.

Carers and teachers have to be careful to ensure that the language they use and the way they use it is clear and unambiguous. When trying to communicate with someone who has problems with social communication, it is important to choose words carefully and not just chatter away. Short, simple phrases with emphasis on key words are more effective. You must also LISTEN carefully to learn how the client uses language.

You might even take the time and trouble to carry out a word audit for each person with an autism This involves listing key words and phrases that the person definitely understands. It also involves identifying alternative ways of expressing something where there is a difficulty with your preferred words. This will enable you to plan and script your verbal communication to make it more effective.

An example of how this works is the experience of David (true story, name changed) who had a job in a bakery, where hygiene was important. He enjoyed the work and was good at it but was on course to lose his job because when he was asked to "Go and wash your hands please", he would wander off looking confused and not wash his hands. A word audit was carried out and it was discovered that David associated the word *wash* with *laundry*. So when he was asked to go and wash his hands he went off looking for a washing machine instead of the wash hand basin. The alternative "Clean your hands please" elicited the correct response.

In the first request the *key word* was 'wash', after which David took no further meaning from the sentence. The word audit identified a *key phrase* which David was able to respond appropriately to. He kept his job because someone in authority was prepared to listen and to change their behaviour.

REMEMBER

Keep speech simple, to the point, and appropriate to the individual.

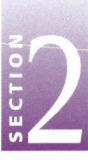

NON-VERBAL COMMUNICATION

Notes

GIVING WORDS MEANING

When two or more people talk together they use more than just words to communicate. Words can be given a variety of meanings by the non-verbal (body language) communication that is given at the same time. Also, tone of voice can greatly affect the message and how it is received.

We all know how a smile or a frown can alter the meaning of a few words and give reassurance or cause concern. One of the problems of speaking to someone on a telephone is that you cannot see the non-verbal language they are using as they speak. In a situation like that we have to rely on the tone of voice of the person speaking to help us judge what they mean.

What do the following words mean? It may help you to read the instructions on how they should be read and then say them out loud:

"Oh yes, *very good*" (said with a smile and emphasis placed on the words "*very good*")

"Oh, yes *very* good" (said in a sneering tone, with a despairing facial expression and with emphasis on the word "*very*").

Just as we need to make sure we use words accurately when we write them down, we also need to control our body language and our tone of voice when we are speaking. If we look or sound miserable when we are talking about something, people might be expected to assume it is not good. If we talk about something whilst lolling in a chair and using a tone of voice that sounds casual, then people may assume that the matter is not to be taken seriously.

It is very important to be calm and consistent at all times, and be careful to remember that you might well be communicating mixed messages to people with autism, whilst at the same time mistakenly assuming that they fully understand.

COMMUNICATION GUIDELINES FOR ADDRESSING PEOPLE WITH AUTISM

LISTENING

People with autism have difficulty in expressing themselves and especially with explaining how they feel and what their needs are. The words they use may not always say exactly what they mean – some may just be repeating phrases they have learned.

Listen carefully to the words used and their possible meaning.

Do not assume that the person necessarily understands the meaning of the words s/he has used.

Some people with autism make up words and sayings, some quite creative and amusing but not always making sense to you. Learn what these words or sayings mean for the person using them.

Some of what people say may sound strange and inappropriate, but do not assume that there is no meaning attached to it.

Ask colleagues about things that are said to you but which you do not understand.

Notes

TALKING

People with autism have the greatest difficulty in following a conversation. Too many words, spoken too fast will cause confusion. They need time to consider what is said to them and the meaning of it. They have difficulty in interpreting facial expression and body language and may confuse alarm or urgency with anger. They take what you say literally.

Be prepared to modify your normal behaviour in conversation for the benefit of clients.

When addressing clients, get into the habit of using their name first.

Do not use many words when a few will do – avoid overloading clients with chatter.

Think carefully about the message you wish to convey, before you speak.

Focus on key words and cut down on the blather. Keep it simple, precise and to the point.

Try to use language, words and tone of voice consistently.

Avoid puns, jokes and word play. Do not be ironic or sarcastic. Avoid being untruthful.

Be very clear and explicit when giving instructions – keep it simple and precise.

BEHAVIOUR

People with autism cannot imagine what might be going on in your mind. They do not understand why your behaviour might change from day to day or even minute by minute. They will have difficulty in judging how appropriate a behaviour is in any given situation.

Maintain a consistent, predictable approach with people on a day-to-day basis.

Try not to let your personal feelings affect the way you behave.

Leave your personal problems at the front door; do not inflict them on the clients.

Do not indulge in 'horse play'; remember that your fooling around is likely to be copied in circumstances which are inappropriate and dangerous.

REMEMBER

Remember that you are a role model – be a good one.

WORKSHEET

5

COMMUNICATION

Answer the following questions:

1. What difficulties do people with autism have with conversation?

_____

_____

_____

_____

2. What difficulties do people with autism have in understanding social situations?

_____

_____

_____

_____

3. In what ways might you be able to help the people with autism with communication?

_____

_____

_____

_____

4. How might you have to modify your own behaviour to help people with autism?

_____

_____

_____

_____

Notes

WORKING WITH THE TRIAD

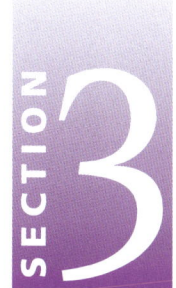

SOME WAYS IN WHICH AUTISM IS DISPLAYED

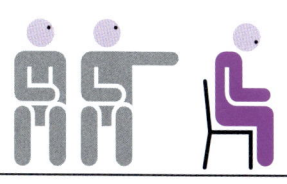

ISOLATED

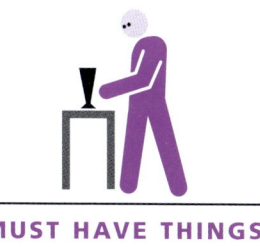

MUST HAVE THINGS EXACTLY IN PLACE

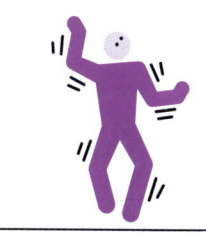

BIZARRE BEHAVIOUR AND MANNERISMS

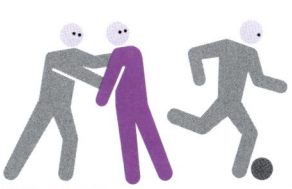

JOINS IN ONLY IF OTHERS INSIST

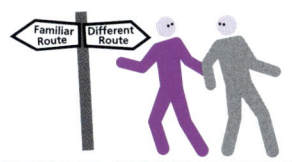

CHANGE IS NOT WELCOME

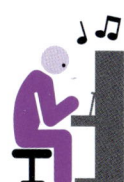

MAY HAVE ISOLATED AREA OF ABILITY

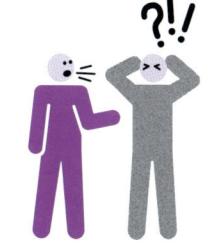

ONE-SIDED INTERACTION

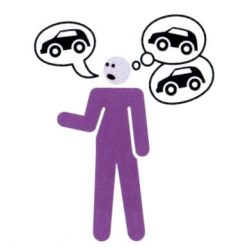

TALKS AND THINKS INCESSANTLY ABOUT ONE TOPIC

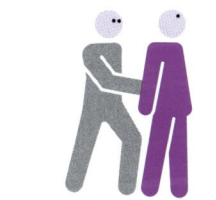

DISPLAYS INDIFFERENCE

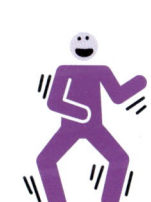

INAPPROPRIATE LAUGHING OR GIGGLING

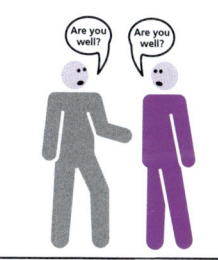

ECHOLALIC – COPIES SPEECH PARROT FASHION

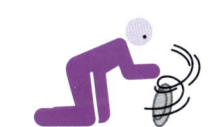

USES OBJECTS WITHOUT AWARENESS OF THEIR REAL USE

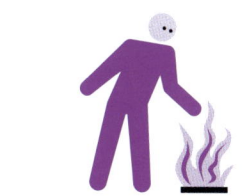

UNAWARE OF COMMON DANGERS

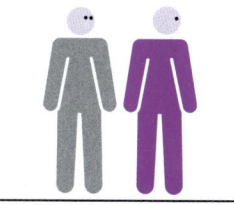

NO EYE CONTACT

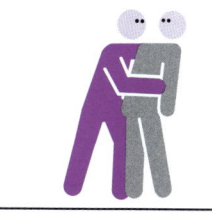

APPROACHES PEOPLE INAPPROPRIATELY

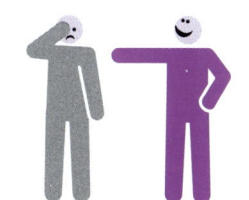

MAY DISPLAY INAPPROPRIATE EMOTIONS

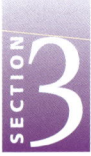

IMPAIRMENT OF SOCIAL INTERACTION

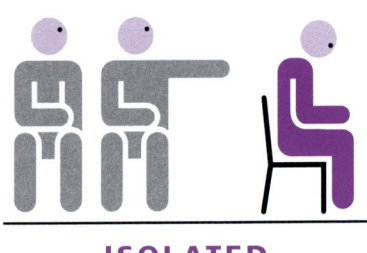

ISOLATED

Range of Impairment:
Aloof
Passive
Active but Odd

You may have noticed that some of the people you are working with tend to be isolated from others, even when they are in the same room. Perhaps they prefer to sit or stand apart from other people; make few attempts to relate to others; seem to become uncomfortable or upset when other people try to relate to them.

This does not necessarily mean that the aloof person does not want to relate to others, it means that they do not know how to do so. Rather than growing up with lots of memories of successful relationships and an understanding that social interaction is enjoyable, some people with autism have memories of all the times they failed to understand other people and were confused, made to feel uncomfortable or were frightened by the behaviour and the words used by other people.

They could not understand what was expected of them or how to engage in mutually beneficial relationships. Rather than keep on trying to cope with experiences that confuse and frighten them, some people with autism learn to try to ignore other people as much as they can. This is a coping mechanism which has the negative effect of isolating the individual from others.

 EXERCISE

Think about occasions in your life when you have felt uncomfortable in the company of others or in certain social situations. For instance, you might have had to attend a social gathering where you did not know anybody. When you got there you may have found that you had little in common with them or have felt excluded by them. You may have experienced feelings of confusion, trepidation or even fear.

Do you try to spend more time in these situations, or less time?

If you cannot entirely avoid them, how do you try to cope when you have to be exposed to them?

REMEMBER

Aloof behaviour does not necessarily mean that the person with autism dislikes you or the other people around them.

Aloof behaviour is probably an indication that the person has had difficulty in understanding other people and has found it more comfortable to ignore them.

If we want to help socially isolated people we need to behave in a way that shows them that they can understand what we are doing, and what we want them to do.

Our behaviour includes both physical actions and language. If you are to help people understand your actions and your language, it is your responsibility to behave and speak clearly in a way they can understand.

Notes

WAYS OF HELPING

- Do not force people who have difficulty in relating to others into crowded situations, particularly where they will have to cope with physical contact, and with lots of people talking.

- Keep the behaviour that you display to the person the same each day. If you are naturally calm this will be fairly easy. If you are an excitable person, learn to control yourself.

- Do not stand too close to the person or force them to accept unnecessary physical contact with you.

- When you speak to the person start by saying their name. Keep sentences and phrases short. Give time for the person to understand what you have said before you add more words.

- Do not start contact by asking the person a question, or demanding that they acknowledge your presence.

- Keep your voice at a normal volume. We often speak louder when we are trying to encourage someone. The person is either unlikely to understand what loud speech means, or may misunderstand and assume you are angry.

- Do not assume that your physical gestures and facial expressions will be understood by the person.

Notes

....

- Do not always use speech when offering companionship to the person. If they have difficulty understanding what you say, they may enjoy your silent presence far more than if you always insist on 'having a chat'.

- Create situations where the person needs to interact with someone else, eg: massage/aromatherapy; carrying something together; interactive games; helping with a task. Make sure the person experiences success by giving praise and rewards.

- Do not become impatient if the person does not respond quickly. It will take time for them to change their ideas about the value of responding to other people.

▶ TASK

Select one client who appears to try to remain apart from others or seems to prefer it if people do not try to relate to them. Use Worksheet 6 to describe their behaviour and to draw up a plan for working to help them find social contact more rewarding. Use as many of the points above as you feel can be applied to the person you have selected.

Your plan will be specific to one client only, as it would not necessarily be appropriate for anybody else who has a similar difficulty. Consider how you might have to adapt this approach to help other clients.

When you have completed the plan discuss it with your study supervisor. Remember that you should not start using your plan at this stage. If you feel that your ideas might help the client, talk the plan through with your line manager.

WORKSHEET
6 | WORKING WITH THE TRIAD

Description of present behaviour

_____

_____

_____

_____

_____

_____

_____

_____

_____

_____

_____

_____

Plan for helping change that behaviour

_____

_____

_____

_____

_____

_____

_____

_____

_____

_____

_____

_____

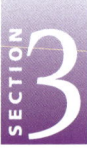
IMPAIRMENT OF SOCIAL INTERACTION

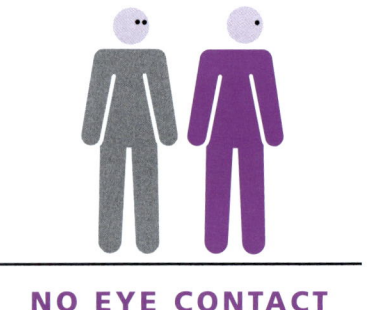

NO EYE CONTACT

Range of Impairment:
Aloof
Passive
Active but Odd

You may have noticed that some of your clients have a degree of difficulty in making eye contact with you when you talk to them, or when you are trying to gain their attention. Avoiding eye contact is very common in people who feel socially isolated and is also seen to varying degrees amongst people who feel awkward in the presence of others.

Some people actually develop such a fear of eye contact that it becomes a phobia. This extreme fear of eye contact is known as scopophobia. It does not only affect people with autism but can affect people in all walks of life.

Avoidance of eye contact is one of the behaviours displayed by people with autism that we should find fairly easy to understand and also to experience for ourselves. You will probably have experienced the embarrassment of 'locking' eyes with someone else at some point in your life. The social rules for eye contact are very complex, the length of time it is acceptable to hold eye contact depends on a number of factors, such as how well you know a person, the social situation, etc.

 EXERCISE

Take the time to observe each of the clients you work with regularly.

How many of them do not make eye contact at all?

How many make eye contact occasionally?

How many make limited eye contact?

Think about holding eye contact yourself. When do you feel awkward?

Try holding eye contact with your study supervisor – how long before you both burst out laughing? Why do you laugh, what purpose does laughter have in this situation?

REMEMBER

Failure to make eye contact does not mean that the person is ignoring you.

People who are not looking at you will not be able to understand any meaning you put into your facial expression (eg smile/frown) or your body language (eg pointing).

Those who make too much eye contact make others feel uncomfortable and embarrassed.

Forcing people to make eye contact when they do not find this to be easy will make them uncomfortable about all the social contact you are making with them.

Judging the appropriate time to hold eye contact with another is a complex social skill which we take for granted.

WAYS OF HELPING

- Say the person's name before expecting them to look at you.

- Teach the person to look in your direction when they hear you say their name. Do not bombard them with speech as soon as they look at you. First smile, then continue with short phrases. If the person is not distressed by physical contact you may place your fingers gently on one side of their chin, using very gentle pressure to show them which way they should look.

- Expect the person to look towards you when they want to communicate with you, either through their signs, gestures, or spoken language.

- Insisting that the person looks into your eyes to show they are listening to you may make them feel uncomfortable. Ask them to look at you instead and to watch you while you talk to them.

- If the person is able to understand, it can be helpful to show them how you look at them – use a diagram to show how your eyes move around someone's face and shoulders, occasionally moving to their arms/hands if they make a gesture, and then back to their face.

- Use drama, games and role play to help people understand why they need to watch other people who are interacting with them. A simple approach, suitable for intellectually able people with autism, is to play charades, using gestures to indicate the meaning, which they must guess. Do not make your subject too difficult.

SECTION 3

Notes

TASK

Select one client who does not make eye contact during social interaction, or who has some difficulty in doing so.

Use Worksheet 7 to describe their behaviour, and to draw up a plan for working to help them give a better appearance of paying attention to those who are communicating with them. Use as many of the points above as you feel can be applied to the person you have selected.

Your plan will be specific to one client only, as it would not necessarily be appropriate for anybody else who has a similar difficulty. Consider how you might have to adapt this approach to help other clients.

Remember that you should not try to implement your plan without the agreement of your line manager and the rest of the staff team.

WORKSHEET
7 | WORKING WITH THE TRIAD

Description of present behaviour

_____

_____

_____

_____

_____

_____

_____

_____

_____

_____

_____

Plan for helping change that behaviour

_____

_____

_____

_____

_____

_____

_____

_____

_____

_____

_____

_____

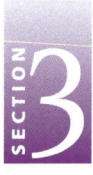

IMPAIRMENT OF SOCIAL INTERACTION

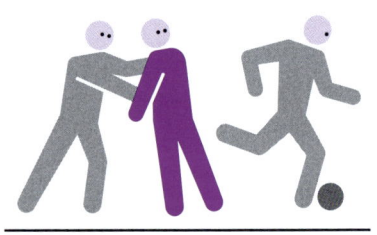

JOINS IN ONLY IF OTHERS INSIST

Range of Impairment:
Aloof
Passive
Active but Odd

During your work with the client group you may have come across people who are best described as being socially 'passive'. They do not seem to be very interested in what is going on around them, and if left to themselves either do nothing, or follow a very limited range of repetitive activities.

In terms of social activity, passive people are usually willing to cooperate with you when you insist on relating to them but rarely take the initiative of starting social interaction themselves.

Passive people may not think to get a drink when they are thirsty but will wait until you suggest that they do so. Similarly they may be too hot but not remove their coat unless you suggest it.

When you know that a person is usually socially active but find them becoming passive in certain situations, you need to be aware that they may be feeling insecure, lacking the confidence to be themselves.

Problems with understanding what is required of them can make people appear to be passive. The person who does not realise you have spoken to them will appear to be passive as they have not responded to you.

Equally someone who has fully understood what is required of them may choose not to respond, or may respond in part only, going to where you asked them to go, but not doing what you wanted them to do when they got there.

 EXERCISE

Observe the group of clients you work with and decide:

How many only join in activity when staff provide the motivation?

How many are usually active but appear passive if they are confused?

How many could best be described as preferring to do nothing at all?

REMEMBER

You should not assume that the lack of response of passive people means that they do not want to join in. They may not understand what you want them to do.

Passive people often need a high degree of staff support, as they need someone with them to provide the motivation to be active.

Passive people are not choosing this way of life but suffer from the triad of impairments. We should not leave them to do nothing.

WAYS OF HELPING

- Do not try to force passive people to be socially active. If they are distressed by being forced you may simply teach them to withdraw even further when people try to relate to them. Work with passive people is about encouraging, never forcing.

- Take responsibility for providing passive people with the motivation they need. Do things with them, not for them.

- Make sure that each person has an effective way in which they can communicate what they want. Some people find speaking difficult but might be willing to learn a sign, or learn to point to a picture, to show what it is that they want.

- Make sure that each person has an effective and acceptable way of saying 'no'. Sometimes people display passive behaviour as a way of indicating that they do not want to get involved in something. This is hard for us to understand. What we need is the word 'no', or a shake of the head, or a sign or symbol for 'no'.

- Regularly include the person's favourite activities in your work with them. Build up a wider range of activity based on what they respond to most actively, eg if the person is enthusiastic about eating food, get them involved in preparing it and shopping for it as well.

- Explain so that the person can understand what an activity requires of them, and for how long it will last. Sometimes we forget that a client may fail to understand that a request to "Come and do some cleaning with me", for instance, is not going to involve them in hard physical work for all the hours remaining in the day. What we should say is "Come and do some cleaning with me and then we will…" (have a coffee, lunch, watch TV, or whatever is appropriate).

Notes

Notes
....

TASK

Identify the person you see as being the most passive of all the clients you work with. If you are not sure who this is, observe the group over a few days before making your selection.

Use Worksheet 8 to describe the way in which the person displays their passive behaviour and to draw up a plan for gently encouraging them to become more socially active.

Your plan will be specific to one client only, as it would not necessarily be appropriate for anybody else who has a similar difficulty. Consider how you might have to adapt this approach to help other clients.

Remember that you should not try to implement your plan without the agreement of your line manager and the rest of the staff team.

WORKSHEET

8 | WORKING WITH THE TRIAD

Description of present behaviour

_____
_____
_____
_____
_____
_____
_____
_____
_____
_____
_____

Plan for helping change that behaviour

_____
_____
_____
_____
_____
_____
_____
_____
_____
_____
_____
_____
_____

IMPAIRMENT OF SOCIAL INTERACTION

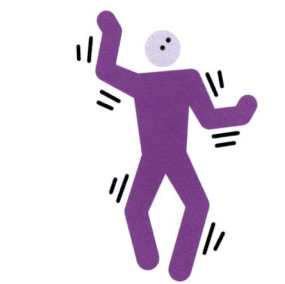

BIZARRE BEHAVIOUR AND MANNERISMS

Range of Impairment:
Aloof
Passive
Active but Odd

Odd and unusual body movements are very common amongst children with autism. As those children grow to adulthood some of them continue to make the same movements, and these can mark them out to other people as being 'different'.

There are two reasons why the children adopt these odd movements. Some children with autism are believed to twirl and rock their bodies to gain sensations and feelings they feel comforted by. Very similar behaviour is sometimes seen in young children who are both blind and deaf. In their case these odd behaviours are believed to be caused by the children lacking other forms of stimulation, ie sight and sound.

The second reason may be the high incidence of repetitive behaviour that is found amongst people with autism. You will be looking in depth at the reasons for repetitive behaviours in Section 4 of the workbook.

 EXERCISE

Observe the clients you are working with and make a note of any movements of body, limbs, or head, that seem to be unusual, either because they just look odd or because they are repeated over and over again.

Can you see any reason for these odd movements? For example, do they occur when the person is not stimulated by other events? Do they occur when the person seems to be anxious or upset?

Think about your own behaviour. Do you make any repetitive movements when you are bored or anxious, such as drumming your fingers, tapping your feet, flicking a pen, etc?

Make notes to assist you in discussing these behaviours with your study supervisor.

40

REMEMBER

If the odd body movements are a form of self-stimulation they will tend to occur when the person is what we might think of as being bored.

If the odd or unusual body movements are repetitive they are more likely to occur when the person is feeling anxious. Anxiety is often caused by the person not understanding what is going on or knowing what is coming next in their lives.

An unusual body movement may not be something that matters very much, particularly when the person is in the privacy of their own home.

Sometimes a particular odd way of moving can cause strain on the body, leading to health problems in later life, eg walking continually on tip-toe can cause shortening of the tendon that runs from the calf muscle to the heel. Once the tendon has shortened the foot can never be placed flat.

WAYS OF HELPING

- Often bizarre and unusual mannerisms have been used by the person for many years. Do not get impatient with them or criticise them for making these movements. They can no more help making them than you can help tapping your fingers, fiddling with your hair, or any of the other mannerisms that you think of as being normal because many people have them.

- If the person carries out their unusual body movements because they are feeling bored it can help them if they are invited to join in an activity that they find interesting.

- If the odd behaviour occurs when the person is anxious, offering them something interesting to do may not help them. Anxiety is often caused by not knowing what to do. A new activity, or one the person is not sure about, may make them feel even more anxious. Think through what might be worrying the person and reassure them if you can. If in doubt offer them familiar activities that you know they understand and can do.

- With intellectually-able people you may be able to gently discuss their unusual body movements with them perhaps using photographs or a video of their behaviour to help them understand what you mean. Point out that their behaviour makes them look unusual. Ask them to compare their odd movements to the behaviour of other people in the community.

Notes

Notes

- If you are asking someone to remember not to display their unusual or bizarre movements when out in the community, reassure them about where and when it is alright to do that. Usually this will be in the privacy of their own home.

- If possible teach the person something else to do when they feel bored, or anxious. If you teach them to tap their fingers instead of rocking backwards and forwards in a chair, remember not to criticise them for tapping their fingers later on.

> ### ▶ TASK
>
> Select one person who displays an unusual or odd way of moving and use Worksheet 9 to:
>
> > (i) describe the behaviour
> >
> > (ii) say when it usually occurs.
>
> Decide if the behaviour might cause the person to be thought of as being odd when they go out into the community, and suggest ways in which you might try to help them change the behaviour.
>
> Your plan will be specific to one client only, as it would not necessarily be appropriate for anybody else who has a similar difficulty. Consider how you might have to adapt this approach to help other clients.
>
> Remember that you should not try to implement your plan without the agreement of your line manager and the rest of the staff team.

WORKSHEET
9

WORKING WITH THE TRIAD

Description of present behaviour

_____

_____

_____

_____

_____

_____

_____

_____

_____

_____

_____

Plan for helping change that behaviour

_____

_____

_____

_____

_____

_____

_____

_____

_____

_____

_____

_____

_____

IMPAIRMENT OF SOCIAL INTERACTION

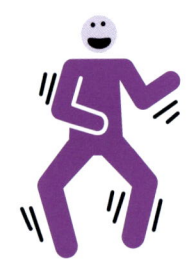

INAPPROPRIATE LAUGHING OR GIGGLING

Range of Impairment:
Aloof
Passive
Active but Odd

Sometimes people with autism burst out laughing, or start giggling, for no apparent reason. When asked what they are laughing at they often do not seem to know.

It is possible that they simply do not choose to share the idea that has amused them. We might understand this if we knew what they were thinking about when they started to laugh.

Another explanation is that the laughter is not always associated with amusing events or ideas. It is often an automatic response to feelings other than mirth, which provides a release of nervous tension. Laughter is sometimes used to cover up social gaffes, such as when somebody says something silly and, realising this, tries to pass it off as a joke.

 EXERCISE

Spend some time watching people around you, both at work and in your social life. Make a mental note of the times and situations where you see people laughing when there has been no joke.

Watch how people behave:

when they are embarrassed

when they are nervous

when they think they have been foolish

when something takes them by surprise

when they know they cannot do something properly.

What did you see?

What function does laughter serve other than to express amusement?

REMEMBER

Laughter is a response to many different types of feeling, not just amusement.

A person with autism is likely to be ill at ease in social situations and to feel that they are making social gaffes.

The person with autism may not know the words to describe the feeling that made them laugh or giggle.

When you laugh, people do not immediately demand to know what you are laughing at.

Notes

WAYS OF HELPING

- Do not automatically demand an explanation for inappropriate laughter.

- Do not become impatient when people laugh inappropriately. If the laughter is caused by nervousness, your impatience will just make the person even more nervous.

- If this behaviour occurs frequently keep a record of when it occurs, and what was happening immediately before the person started to laugh. This will help you decide what is causing the behaviour.

- Remember that it is perfectly normal for people to laugh or giggle in response to many types of feelings. If the behaviour seems to be linked to nervousness or anxiety then offer the person more reassurance on more occasions during every day.

- The behaviour may be linked to mild shock or surprise, perhaps because the person was not concentrating and is taken by surprise when people touch or talk to them. Remember always to say their name before you start to interact with them. Give them time to hear their name and realise that something is about to happen, before you continue.

- Where the behaviour might be linked to the person knowing that they cannot do what is asked of them (this is called defensive laughter, something that you might remember from school, when the teacher asked you a question you could not answer), review the individual programme plans that have been written for the person. They may be asking too much of the person and may need simplifying.

Notes

TASK

If you have a client who laughs or giggles inappropriately, carry out observations of him/her over the next week. Record when you see the behaviour and what was happening immediately before the laughter started.

Use Worksheet 10 to describe the behaviour and the results of your observations. Decide if the behaviour needs to be changed, or if it would be more appropriate for staff to simply accept it. If change is necessary, write down how you might approach the situation, using as many of the above points as seem to be relevant.

Your plan will be specific to one client only, as it would not necessarily be appropriate for anybody else who has a similar difficulty. Consider how you might have to adapt this approach to help other clients.

Remember that you should not try to implement your plan without the agreement of your line manager and the rest of the staff team.

WORKSHEET 10

WORKING WITH THE TRIAD

Description of present behaviour

_____

_____

_____

_____

_____

_____

_____

_____

_____

_____

_____

_____

Plan for helping change that behaviour

_____

_____

_____

_____

_____

_____

_____

_____

_____

_____

_____

_____

IMPAIRMENT OF SOCIAL INTERACTION

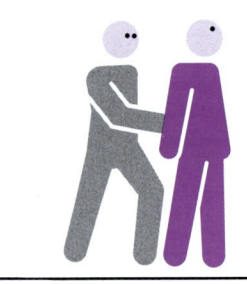

DISPLAYS INDIFFERENCE

Range of Impairment:
Aloof
Passive
Active but Odd

Not all displays of social indifference indicate an aloof or passive response.

In the terminology used to describe the social relating skills of people with autism, 'aloof' means that the person is unlikely to start nor may even welcome social contact with others. Passive people are those who do not try to start social contact but will accept social advances made towards them by other people. The category of active but odd describes people who are trying to make social contact with others but who have limited, and often mistaken ideas of how this should be done.

You might expect that a display of social indifference by a person with autism automatically places them in the socially aloof or passive categories. Whilst this may be true, you must avoid making automatic assumptions.

 EXERCISE

Select those people you work with who display social indifference towards you and other people. This indifference may take the form of ignoring you when you speak, treating you like an object, moving away when you stand/sit next to them or having to be physically coaxed into joining in activities with other people.

Spend the next week observing this group of people as closely as you can and answer the following questions for each person:

Does the person display any inappropriate behaviour that means staff have to pay them attention?

Does the person seem to have difficulty with any task, requiring staff to assist them?

Does the person display any other form of behaviour that seems to be deliberately used to attract the attention of other people?

Does the person display any other form of behaviour that makes it necessary for people to pay them extra attention?

At the end of the exercise decide which of the people you have selected are socially Aloof, Passive, or Active but Odd. Discuss your decision with your line manager.

Notes
....

REMEMBER

People with autism have an impairment of their social-relating skills. This does not mean that all people with autism are antisocial. Not knowing how to relate to others is not the same thing as not wanting to relate to them.

WAYS OF HELPING

- When clients are unresponsive towards you, do not allow yourself to think that they dislike you. The judgements you are used to making in your own social life should not be applied to your professional relationships with people with autism.

- Do not force people with autism into situations where they must interact with others. Any anxiety they feel will have been caused by you. Any inappropriate behaviour they display will be your responsibility.

- Do not assume that people with autism dislike social contact. Get to know them and see how they wish to relate to others.

- Be sensitive to the amount of space a person with autism may wish to have between themselves and other people. A person who cannot cope with having you stand next to them may be able to enjoy your company if you are some distance away.

- Do not bombard people with autism with words. Relaxing companionship can exist without continual speech. Instead of talking all the time, face towards the person, looking directly at them from time to time, to show that you are paying them attention.

- Get to know what things interest the person and build up their trust in you by showing interest in the same thing where possible.

Notes
....

- If the person has an unacceptable way of seeking your attention, deal with this by giving them your attention before they have to use their inappropriate behaviour to remind you that they need some of your time.

- Be rewarding to the person. Praise them. Make them feel that you value them. Smile at them. Above all behave and speak as though you like them. How else can they gain the confidence to relate to you?

> **TASK**
>
> Select one of the people you identified as being socially unresponsive. Use Worksheet 11 to describe their present social behaviour. Describe how you might set about encouraging the person to become more socially responsive, using as many of the above points as seem to be relevant to the person concerned.
>
> Your plan will be specific to one client only, as it would not necessarily be appropriate for anybody else who has a similar difficulty. Consider how you might have to adapt this approach to help other clients.
>
> Remember that you should not try to implement your plan without the agreement of your line manager and the rest of the staff team.

WORKSHEET
11   WORKING WITH THE TRIAD

Description of present behaviour

_____
_____
_____
_____
_____
_____
_____
_____
_____
_____
_____
_____

Plan for helping change that behaviour

_____
_____
_____
_____
_____
_____
_____
_____
_____
_____
_____
_____

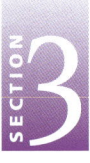
IMPAIRMENT OF SOCIAL INTERACTION

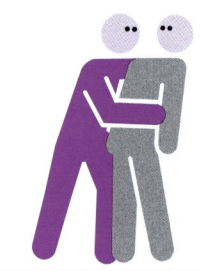

APPROACHES PEOPLE INAPPROPRIATELY

Although the common perception of people with autistic spectrum disorders is that they tend to shun contact with others, a significant number actively seek it out. Often though, the way they approach people is perceived as odd and inappropriate. For instance they may start an encounter with an intrusive question or unfortunate comment, or even inappropriate physical contact. Such approaches are likely to cause the recipient some discomfort or embarrassment. Being asked one's age or receiving comment about one's appearance by way of an introductory remark is usually considered rude. Although eye contact is important, staring relentlessly is disconcerting and challenging. Approaching too closely or grabbing hold of someone can be seen as aggressive (and even painful!).

People with autism who approach others inappropriately tend to fall into the 'Active but Odd' range of the impairment. Such people are often sociable, enjoy the company of others and their approaches are just their way of being friendly. Unfortunately their behaviour is often seen as intrusive and off-putting, and can result in a rebuff. This can be upsetting and frustrating for the person with autism and may sometimes result in a distress reaction or outburst. Sometimes the inevitable response to an inappropriate approach is expected or even sought and is rewarding to the person with autism.

It is important that people with autism are enabled to achieve success with their social encounters. Rather than allow the person to become socially isolated we can teach a set of simple social skills to replace the inappropriate ones. We can also intervene in social encounters to model appropriate behaviours that the person with autism can copy. However, it is important to be aware that we use our social judgement when approaching others and adopt a variety of behaviours depending on the situation. People with autism will not have the ability to use sophisticated social judgement so will need a safe strategy that will serve them in a number of situations.

EXERCISE

Think about occasions when you have to meet and greet people. Sometimes they will be familiar to you, sometimes they will be complete strangers. How does your behaviour change in different circumstances and with different people. For instance, would you greet a prospective employer at an interview in the same way as you would your best friend at a party? Probably not!

Think also about how people approach you under different circumstances. For instance, would you be happy that a complete stranger grabbed your arm or put their hand on your knee to keep your attention or emphasise a point?

Think about eye contact. How do you ensure that those you are speaking to are given enough eye contact to encourage them but not so much as to make them feel uncomfortable?

If you were only allowed to have one method of meeting and greeting people, which would be safe, non-offensive, not over-familiar but open and friendly, how would you choose to behave?

Notes
....

REMEMBER

Active but Odd social behaviour is exhibited because the person engaging in it has a limited behavioural repertoire. They are unlikely to be behaving in such a way to deliberately make others feel uncomfortable.

People with autism do not always learn from experience alone because of the difficulties they have with generalising their experiences. Therefore, although their odd behaviour does not have the desired effect they will not modify it on their own.

People with autism can become so used to the response they get or the rejection following their inappropriate response that, to them, it becomes the norm and provides its own reward or reassurance. They might even repeat or increase the behaviour to ensure that the expected response is forthcoming.

The person who exhibits inappropriate meeting and greeting behaviour is as likely to become just as socially isolated as the one who is socially aloof.

Notes

....

Behaviours can be learned if someone is prepared to teach. For inappropriate behaviours to be reduced, more appropriate ones must be taught to take their place.

People with autistic spectrum disorders will not be able to exercise sophisticated social judgement in the way the rest of us take for granted, because of the nature of their disability. They will not have the choice of alternative appropriate behaviours to try out as the occasion demands.

WAYS OF HELPING

- Do not criticise the person who is trying their best to engage with others but getting it wrong.

- Remember that you are a role model. Demonstrate appropriate behaviour in the workplace and avoid the temptation to be over-familiar with people you know well.

- Teach a 'failsafe' meeting and greeting routine, which will serve for most situations and that will not repel the person they wish to approach. An outstretched hand serves to encourage appropriate physical contact (the handshake) and also to ensure appropriate distance (arm's length). The routine needs to be learned by rote and reinforced with verbal and physical prompts until it becomes automatic.

- Be aware when a social gaffe is likely and be prepared to intervene by making an introduction. You may use your physical presence to forestall inappropriate physical distance and/or contact.

- Model the behaviour yourself by using it at times when you have not seen the person for a day or two, for instance when you come on duty or meet them in the street. Ensure that all your colleagues do the same thing.

- Get the person you are supporting to practise the skill in role modelling sessions. You play the part of the person to be greeted and allow your student/client to practise their appropriate greeting behaviour until they get it right consistently.

- A verbal cue might be useful for the stranger too. Saying something like "This is Martin, he would like to shake your hand", might be useful for both parties and trigger the behaviour.

- Always acknowledge a successful encounter with praise and encouragement.

- Be prepared for the client to appear rather formal and stilted in some circumstances with their 'failsafe' routine. They might even use it too much but this is likely to be better than inappropriate contact and touching. At least it will be reasonable, appropriate, non-threatening and acceptable.

TASK

Select one client who approaches other people inappropriately. Use Worksheet 12 to describe the undesired behaviours and draw up a plan for replacing them with more appropriate ones.

Your plan will be specific to one client. Remember that you are not trying to teach social judgement. You are trying to teach a 'failsafe' meeting and greeting routine to replace inappropriate approach behaviour. The client may eventually develop a repertoire of skills from which they can select the most appropriate for the occasion, but for now you are at stage one.

Remember that you should not try to implement your plan without the agreement and co-operation of your line manager and the rest of the staff team.

WORKING WITH THE TRIAD

Description of present behaviour

_____

_____

_____

_____

_____

_____

_____

_____

_____

_____

_____

Plan for helping change that behaviour

_____

_____

_____

_____

_____

_____

_____

_____

_____

_____

_____

_____

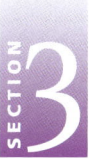
IMPAIRMENT OF SOCIAL COMMUNICATION

Echolalia and Repetitive Speech

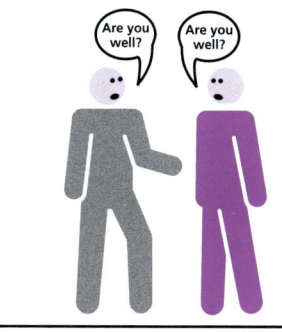

ECHOLALIC – COPIES SPEECH PARROT FASHION

Echolalia can be an instant repetition of the words someone else has just used, or the repetition of words and phrases that have been heard some time before. Some people with echolalia appear to repeat questions they associate with things they want, rather than ask for them themselves. For example when a person with echolalia walks into the room saying "Do you want a cup of tea?" they are copying the words they associate with being offered tea, instead of saying the more normal, "I would like a cup of tea".

In the above example it is easy to see how difficult it must be for people with echolalia to understand our responses. In reply to the words "Do you want a cup of tea?" we might answer "Yes, please" or "No, thank you", as we believe the person is offering us tea. When we understand that the question is not intended to offer something to us but is used by the person in the hope that we will give them a cup of tea, we can see how odd and unhelpful our reply must seem to the person with autism who uses echolalic speech.

EXERCISE

Identify any of the people you are working with who copy the speech of other people, or who repeat set phrases that they may have learnt from other people earlier in their lives.

Observe those people in turn and make a list of the repetitive phrases they use that may be echolalic.

Can you identify any words or phrases that are copies of what other people have said in that situation, rather than the free speech of the person you are observing?

Notes

REMEMBER

People with autism have an impairment of their social communication skills. Echolalic and repetitive speech is just one form that this impairment can take.

We might assume that the person using echolalic speech will learn that this is not an effective way of communicating with other people. This is not true. By always attending to echolalia, we keep on encouraging the person to use this method of communicating.

If we do not teach the correct way of speaking then people with echolalia who want to communicate with us will have no choice but to go on using their echolalic forms of speech.

WAYS OF HELPING

- Do not allow yourself to show feelings of confusion or irritation with people who use echolalic and repetitive speech. If you do react the client will become more certain that this is an effective way of gaining your attention.

- Observe the client to see if they have any free speech which is not echolalic or repetitive. If they do then make sure you pay the client lots of attention every time they speak without repetition or copying.

- If the client has no free speech other than echolalic and repetitive phrases teach them to use single words to name what they are interested in. Reward use of these words by paying instant attention to the client. At the same time totally ignore any echolalic or repetitive speech that the client is habitually using to gain your attention, or to ask for something they want.

- When ignoring echolalic or repetitive speech act as though the words have not been said. Look away from the client to show that you are not responding to them.

- If you get the balance of reward and ignoring right, the client will start to use the new words you have taught, rather than the echolalic or repetitive speech they have used in the past.

- Echolalia sometimes occurs when the client does not understand what is going on. Often this is linked to us using too many words when we speak to the client concerned. Cut down the amount of speech you use. Give time between your sentences for the client to understand what you have said.

- Remember that having other speech going on at the same time as we are speaking can lead to exactly the same effect as the previous point. Think carefully before you talk to the client at the same time as the room is full of other voices speaking from the television or radio. Turn them off before you speak.

Notes

TASK

Select one of the people that you identified as using echolalic or repetitive speech. Use Worksheet 13 to describe the way in which they display this form of impaired social communication skills.

Consider each of the points above and describe how you might go about helping this client to communicate more effectively. Make sure that you clearly show the changes that are going to be required in your behaviour.

Your plan will be specific to one client only, as it would not necessarily be appropriate for anybody else who has a similar difficulty. Consider how you might have to adapt this approach to help other clients.

Remember that you should not try to implement your plan without the agreement of your line manager and the rest of the staff team.

WORKING WITH THE TRIAD

Description of present behaviour

_____

_____

_____

_____

_____

_____

_____

_____

_____

_____

_____

_____

Plan for helping change that behaviour

_____

_____

_____

_____

_____

_____

_____

_____

_____

_____

_____

_____

_____

_____

IMPAIRMENT OF SOCIAL COMMUNICATION

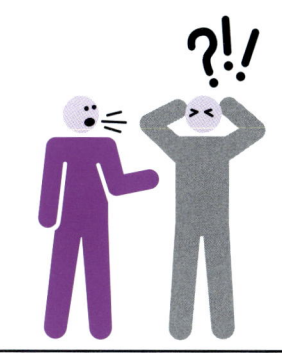

Makes factual comments often irrelevant to the situation
Asks repetitive questions and may ignore answers

ONE-SIDED INTERACTION

In addition to an impairment of social relating skills, people with autism also have difficulty in using their language and communication skills for communication with other people.

Where the clients you are working with have the use of speech, you may have noticed that some of them do not seem to use it to relate to other people. They do not discuss, or debate, or use language to share experiences. Language is not used for social purposes, rather it is used to name their own needs, to make factual statements, or to ask questions about things that may affect them. Often these questions are repetitive, being asked many times each day, regardless of how often you give an answer.

The feeling you may often have is that some of the clients talk at you rather than to you, or with you. Sometimes the client wants you to say little more than those exact words that he or she wishes to hear; others leave no gaps in their speech to allow you a chance to say something. Often, when the client does stop talking, he or she simply wanders away, ignoring what you may try to say to them.

 EXERCISE

Spend the next week observing and listening carefully to the clients that you work with. Make notes and find answers to the following questions:

1. How many have the use of speech?

2. How many use that speech for the kind of social conversations normal to this age group?

3. How many ask repetitive questions, seeming to take little notice of the answers they are given?

4. How many limit their use of speech to saying what they want, or are particularly interested in?

5. How many of them seem to talk at you, rather than with you?

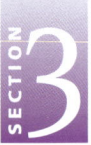
REMEMBER

The social use of language is about interacting with others. Much of what we say is not very important but it does hold us together in social groups. People who use language to talk only about themselves, their interests or what they want, are often seen as selfish, boring people. People with autism do not choose to be like this, they are disabled by an impairment of their social communication skills.

WAYS OF HELPING

- Do not react to the client as though s/he is a selfish, boring person. Negative responses from you will only make the client anxious and even more likely to try to ignore what you and other people say to them.

- If the client asks repetitive questions and expects you to provide exactly the same answer each time, do not confuse them by deliberately giving different answers. This can cause so much anxiety that it could be taken to be a form of mental cruelty and emotional abuse. Anxiety also has the effect of making the client ask their question more often, exactly the opposite to what you should be trying to achieve.

- Reach agreement with all the staff in your team about exactly how many times staff will answer repetitive questions – three times is probably a reasonable number to start with. Explain to the client that you will only answer them so many times. If they ask the question too many times, ask them to repeat the answer you have given. If the question is repeated yet again, ignore it completely.

- An alternative to the above strategy is to agree with all the members of the staff team exactly what times in the day the client can ask their repetitive questions. At the end of a work session, at meal times, before the client goes to bed, are all equally valid. Do not make the client wait too long when you first start this way of working. If the client asks repetitive questions outside of these times, do not answer the question, but tell them when they can ask it again.

- For other forms of one-sided verbal interaction, explain to the client that you want to say something as well, not just listen to them. Ask them to stop talking when you raise your hand, and listen to you (use another type of clue if the client cannot understand a hand movement). Keep what you say very short to start with and do not try to change the subject. Do not ask a question, as it may discourage the client from continuing. Do not discourage or confuse, you want the client to enjoy having you join in.

- If the client does not respond to the above strategy for dealing with one-sided interaction, try using the method which allows it at certain times of the day only.

Notes
....

TASK

Select one of the people you work with who shows a tendency to make one sided verbal interactions. Use Worksheet 14 to describe the way in which they do this. Consider each of the points above and decide which of them may be helpful in working with the client. Describe how you would go about helping the client to use their verbal skills to communicate in a more socially acceptable way.

Your plan will be specific to one client only, as it would not necessarily be appropriate for anybody else who has a similar difficulty. Consider how you might have to adapt this approach to help other clients.

Remember that you should not try to implement your plan without the agreement of your line manager and the rest of the staff team.

WORKING WITH THE TRIAD

Description of present behaviour

_____

_____

_____

_____

_____

_____

_____

_____

_____

_____

_____

_____

Plan for helping change that behaviour

_____

_____

_____

_____

_____

_____

_____

_____

_____

_____

_____

_____

_____

_____

IMPAIRMENT OF SOCIAL COMMUNICATION

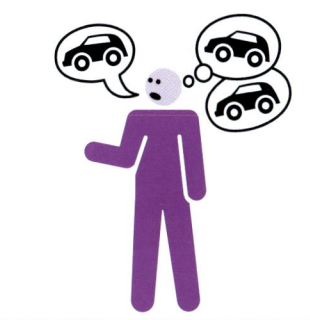

Talks incessantly regardless of the response of others

TALKS AND THINKS INCESSANTLY ABOUT ONE TOPIC

Due to some of the difficulties associated with the impairment of imagination and social understanding (the third element of the Triad of Impairments), many people with autism tend to have very narrow areas of interest. Individuals can become 'obsessed' with one particular topic. They often think about it to the exclusion of everything else that a person of their age might normally have to give some thought to in the course of the day.

While such a person has speech they often talk about their obsession, regardless of the response of other people around them. It is quite common to find signs of this behaviour in people who have no form of disability. You may have friends who sometimes appear to be 'obsessed' with a hobby, a sport, a particular form of music, or perhaps the person they have just fallen in love with. Your friends will also tend to talk about their obsessive interest, more than anything else, so much so that sometimes they can be boring to be with.

People with autism often lack the social understanding required to read the signs that other people give out when they are bored (yawning, glancing at their watch, looking around at other things, fidgeting etc). As they cannot tell when they are boring other people they just go on and on, unaware of the reaction they are causing.

 EXERCISE

Consider the clients you are working with and decide if any of them display this tendency. If so pick one person and listen carefully to them during your work for the next week.

Do they really only talk about their obsessional interest? What else do they talk about, even if it is only for a few moments? What other interests do they have in addition to their obsession? What other activities are they involved in that could be used as something else to talk about?

Notes

....

REMEMBER

It is perfectly normal to want to talk about the thing you know most about. People who have an obsessional interest often do not realise that others are not interested in that particular subject.

People also behave like this when they want to relate to others but do not know what else they can talk about. We often experience this ourselves, for example conversations at social gatherings, such as parties, often cover the same sort of topics, ie the weather, politics, sport, relationships, etc.

WAYS OF HELPING

- Be patient with people who always want to talk about the same thing. We cannot encourage them to learn wider conversational skills at the same time as discouraging them from talking freely about their own interest.

- Remember that the person may not know what else they can talk about. Encourage them to say more about other things in their lives.

- If the person can read, encourage them to look at a daily paper each day, to see what subjects they might be able to talk to other people about. For example, on the day that David Beckham has a new hairstyle many people will respond normally to someone who mentions that fact. Work with the person to help them select some key facts from the newspaper article.

- If the person can understand, teach them the signs that people use when they are getting fed up with listening to the same thing (looking away, yawning, looking at their watch). Teach them to change the subject when they see these signs. If you do not know how to teach these things then set aside sessions of 10-15 minutes each day for a 'game' where the person has to guess what you mean when you make these movements. Offer a reward, one that the person will enjoy, for getting more than half the answers right.

- Encourage the person to talk about other things by clearly showing them that they have your undivided attention when they talk about other topics.

- When the person regularly mentions other topics continue to show your undivided attention for those and start to reduce the amount of attention you give to the obsessional topic of conversation. You can do this by looking away when the conversation turns to the obsession. Or you can use the signs mentioned above, if the person understands what they mean.

- Set aside one time in each day you are at work to allow the person to talk incessantly to you about their obsessional topic. This should be a period of no more than five to ten minutes. Explain to the person that this is when you have the time to listen to them.

- If the person cannot understand or co-operate with any of the above, you may have to simply ask them to stop talking about their obsession. There is a risk that the person will feel socially rejected. You can prevent this by praising them, admiring something about them, making them feel that you are interested in them. Never stop them talking about their obsession and simply allow the interaction between you to end there.

Notes

 TASK

Look at the notes you made about the person you selected as displaying this kind of behaviour. Use Worksheet 15 to describe the way in which they display the tendency to talk incessantly about one topic. Look through the above points and select those that might be of help in changing this behaviour. Describe how you might go about encouraging the person to talk about other topics.

Your plan will be specific to one client only, as it would not necessarily be appropriate for anybody else who has a similar difficulty. Consider how you might have to adapt this approach to help other clients.

Remember that you should not try to implement your plan without the agreement of your line manager and the rest of the staff team.

WORKING WITH THE TRIAD

Description of present behaviour

_____

_____

_____

_____

_____

_____

_____

_____

_____

_____

_____

_____

_____

Plan for helping change that behaviour

_____

_____

_____

_____

_____

_____

_____

_____

_____

_____

_____

_____

_____

IMPAIRMENT OF SOCIAL COMMUNICATION

You may have noticed that some people with autistic spectrum disorders display emotional responses that are inappropriate to the situation. This might be seen as fear of something not generally thought to be frightening, laughter at a personal tragedy, or tears in response to something very trivial. These inappropriate responses not only mark people with autism out as different or odd, but can also cause great offence or upset. If the news of a death in the family is met with howls of laughter or morbid questions, the impression is of not caring or even of malicious intent.

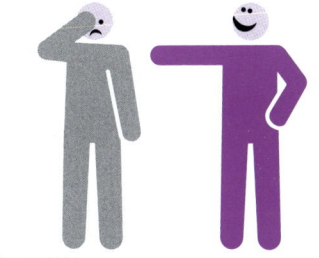

MAY DISPLAY INAPPROPRIATE EMOTIONS

However, the reasons for such inappropriate responses from people with autism are to be found in the condition itself. The ability to conceptualise or imagine the consequences of a situation is lacking. The ability to empathise with another person or to put oneself in their position and imagine how they must be feeling is lacking. The ability to project oneself forward by imagination to anticipate an outcome and behave accordingly is impaired. There is no malice or malign intent, merely a lack of the development of skills (or developmental milestones) that most of us take for granted. Young children are not expected to understand death, the feelings of others or to prepare for the unknown. This is because they are not expected to reach these developmental milestones until a certain age. People with autism might never achieve these milestones and must learn coping strategies instead.

Autism is a disorder of development where certain aspects of the person's skills are impaired. You will have learned that social skills and imaginative ability are particularly affected. Without empathy (theory of mind), the ability to imagine the thoughts and feelings of others, it is very difficult to gauge how to respond appropriately to others. Without imaginative ability it is very difficult to project oneself forward, anticipate consequences and plan appropriate behavioural strategies to meet a situation and thereby reassure oneself. Without this ability any unfamiliar situation is a step into the unknown and, as we are all aware, the unknown is always most frightening.

EXERCISE

Think about how you respond to someone who is upset. How does their emotional state affect you? How do you know what to say and how to say it? How does the gravity of their situation affect your response? How do you know how they are thinking and feeling and what would you be left with if you did not possess this skill?

Think about occasions when you have to prepare for a difficult and frightening experience. For instance, most people have to attend job interviews during their lives and most people find them daunting. How do you prepare for the experience? Do you imagine being in the interview room? Do you imagine the interview panel and what questions they may ask you? Do you rehearse the answers you will give to the likely questions? How will you deal with the questions you have not anticipated? How does all this anticipation and rehearsal reassure you? Suppose that you were not able to go through the process of reassuring yourself that everything would be alright.

Try writing down an explanation of death that would satisfy a young child. How do you explain the concept of life leaving the body, the notion that the flesh remains but the person has gone (and where to)? Consider how difficult it is to explain life in terms other than bodily functions such as heartbeat and breathing. Where has the person gone when their body is still before you? These are questions that have challenged the minds of great philosophers and have spawned religions, yet we have to find an explanation for people who think literally and in concrete terms.

REMEMBER

The inappropriate emotional responses of people with autism are due to impairment in key areas of development.

Laughter in the face of a tragic situation is likely to be a nervous response to a situation that the person with autism does not fully understand and cannot cope with.

People with autism cannot learn empathy in the way most people can. The thoughts and feelings of others are a mystery to them and have to be explained in literal and concrete terms.

Their show of fear of a situation or planned activity might seem silly and dramatic but it is likely to be a response to having to step into the unknown with no idea of the outcome.

People with autistic spectrum disorders will not be able to reassure themselves about a situation by projecting themselves forward in their imaginations to plan their actions in order to ensure a satisfactory (and reassuring) outcome.

WAYS OF HELPING

- Do not criticise the person whose behaviour is insensitive or unfeeling towards others. Take the time to explain the situation in literal, concrete terms. Reassure them that everything is okay but explain that the affected person is upset and why.

- Reassure the person with autism that when someone else is upset, they do not have to worry. Teach them a behavioural strategy for dealing with such situations.

- Remember that you are a role model. Demonstrate appropriate behaviour in the workplace and avoid the temptation to be flippant or inappropriate yourself.

- Do not dismiss the fears and anxieties of people with autism, no matter how trivial they appear to you. Such expressions of emotion are likely to be perfectly genuine. Dismissing them is likely to make things worse. What is required is understanding and reassurance.

- Always ensure that new situations, events or activities are properly explained beforehand and provide reassurance.

- Incorporate theory of mind in social skills training. Although it is not possible to teach empathy or the ability to imagine what others are thinking, it is possible to teach some people with autism that other people have thoughts and feelings and emotions. Also that although these are private and unique to individuals, we can share them if we express them and adopt appropriate behaviours.

Notes

Notes
·····································

- Teach appropriate behaviours. Although it is not possible to teach empathy as such, it is possible to teach people to behave in ways that do not make others feel uncomfortable. For instance, never to laugh when someone is upset.

- Remember that even when people with autism are able to learn how to deal with certain situations, they will continue to need help when they encounter new ones. They will remain unable to judge the thoughts and feelings of others and will continue to have difficulties in unfamiliar circumstances.

IMPAIRMENT OF IMAGINATION AND SOCIAL UNDERSTANDING

Difficulty in generalising concepts and inflexibility of thought

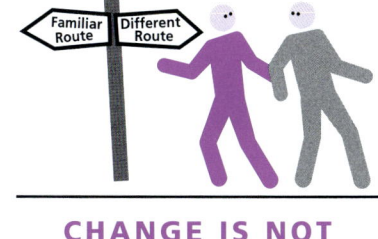

CHANGE IS NOT WELCOME

You may have noticed that some of the clients that you are working with prefer to do familiar things and go to familiar places rather than becoming involved in new experiences. Some of them may appear to be fearful or anxious when they are faced with new experiences.

This liking for the familiar, and dislike of the new and unknown, is caused by an impairment in imagination and social understanding skills (the third element of the Triad of Impairments).

Many people with autism are inflexible in their ideas. Once they have experienced something they expect it to be exactly the same next time. Someone who enjoys going to a cafe for the first time, is quite likely to think that every trip to a cafe will be to that same one where they will sit in the same place and order the same food/drink. They may become distressed when the cafe is redecorated, as the walls are now the 'wrong' colour.

Inflexible thinking is caused by difficulty in generalising ideas. Imagine you are going to a cafe for the first time. After going inside, finding a seat, ordering food and paying for it you would begin to feel more confident that you could go into other cafes in other towns and manage just as well. This is because you can generalise your learning experiences.

A person with autism might learn that they can manage in that cafe but still not believe that they could manage in another cafe. This is because they believe that the look of the cafe, the smell of it, the colour of the seats, the sounds they hear there, are all specific parts of being served with what they want. Naturally no other cafe will have exactly those sights, smells, and sounds – unless it is one of a chain such as Little Chef or McDonald's.

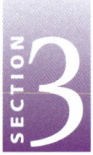

Notes

> ### ▶ EXERCISE
>
> List all the things you do in a typical non-working day. Underline all of those things that you do in a fixed order, and those that might make you feel uncomfortable or irritated if they did not happen as you like them to. Although you can cope with change, do you think that order and repetition have a place in your ability to relax, even on a day off?

REMEMBER

The success of chains of shops and restaurants shows that it is not only people with autism who prefer taking the familiar route. Although we can cope with change many of us prefer to avoid it as much as we can and stick to the familiar – where we feel safe.

WAYS OF HELPING

- Help the people you are working with by giving them experiences in more than one situation, eg do not always shop in the same supermarket whilst training. Use several shops, so that the person has a chance to learn that they can manage in more than one situation.

- Remember that change may always be difficult for the person. When prices of familiar purchases go up they may lose confidence in their ability to shop, or use public transport, etc. Offer support and re-training to rebuild their confidence.

- Be aware of the things that may be an important part of the understanding of a person with autism. The look, the smells, the noise, even the taste, of a particular experience can all be an important part of their understanding and of their confidence that they can manage. When any one of these factors is changed they may need support to help them cope with the change. If we cannot see what has changed, and how important that is, we will not understand their anxiety, or why they are suddenly starting to fail in a situation they used to be able to cope with.

- Be careful when deciding that a person should be able to cope with change. All human beings have some routine in their lives. Without our routines we all feel insecure.

- When you want someone to accept change in their lives always plan that change carefully. Everybody who comes into contact with the person needs to know exactly what is changing, so that they can all give the person the same description of what it is that is about to change.

Notes

- Sometimes people think it is kinder 'not to worry' the person about a change or new experience that is coming up. Instead of being prepared, the person is put through the change/new experience without warning. This is wrong. If people are treated like this they just become anxious that changes can happen without warning at any moment. If you always explain change before it happens then people will be able to trust you when you tell them nothing is changing/new today.

- It can help to rehearse new situations before they happen, eg if the person has to visit the local hospital because of a health problem, take them there before the day of their appointment. Visit the waiting room, if possible have a cup of tea there, so that the hospital becomes known to the person and is associated with positive memories.

TASK

Select one of the people you work with who displays a dislike of change or new experiences. Describe the kind of difficulty they have, and the behaviour that arises from that difficulty. Think through the points above and use Worksheet 16 to write a plan for introducing change or new experience to that person, making use of any of the points that may be helpful to the person.

Your plan will be specific to one client only, as it would not necessarily be appropriate for anybody else who has a similar difficulty. Consider how you might have to adapt this approach to help other clients.

Remember that you should not try to implement your plan without the agreement of your line manager and the rest of the staff team.

WORKING WITH THE TRIAD

Description of present behaviour

_____

_____

_____

_____

_____

_____

_____

_____

_____

_____

_____

_____

Plan for helping change that behaviour

_____

_____

_____

_____

_____

_____

_____

_____

_____

_____

_____

_____

_____

IMPAIRMENT OF IMAGINATION AND SOCIAL UNDERSTANDING

Inflexibility of thought
Repetitive enacting of role

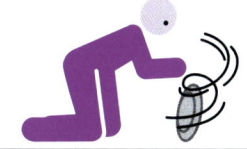

USES OBJECTS WITHOUT AWARENESS OF THEIR REAL USE

Pre-school playgroup staff are frequently amongst the first professional people to notice that a child is displaying the behavioural features of autism. Used to the way in which young children play with toys and handle objects, they rapidly notice the different way in which children with autism handle such objects. A toy car may be held for hours whilst the child repeatedly spins one of the wheels or taps it on the floor. The car is rarely put on its wheels and run along the ground.

Some adults with autism also display a tendency to use objects without understanding their real purpose. Plates may be seen as objects for spinning, rather than as things to put meals on; a broom may be for balancing rather than sweeping; in a craft situation a screwdriver may be seen as being for tapping on the bench, rather than for tightening screws.

We all recognise that some objects have a number of different uses. Most of us will have used a screwdriver as a lever to get the lid off a paint tin at some time in our lives, but we still know what a screwdriver is really meant for.

Some people with autism do not have this ability to be flexible in their understanding of objects. If a screwdriver is for tapping on the table, that is what they use it for. When working in a craft room their first thought on picking up a screwdriver will be to tap with it. Teaching them the real use of the tool has to overcome their own ideas. Often all we can teach is that a screwdriver can also be used for turning screws.

 EXERCISE

Observe the people you are working with and see if you can identify ways in which they display this tendency to use objects without any real understanding of their purpose.

Notes

....

REMEMBER

Just because a person knows the name of an object and can fetch it when asked to do so, it does not mean that they know what it is for and how to use it.

Someone who is using an object for an unusual or inappropriate purpose may think that this is what the object is really for.

This behaviour is not the same as deliberate misuse of tools and objects.

WAYS OF HELPING

- Do not expect people to understand the reasons why we sometimes use objects for a different purpose than the one they were designed for. We really should not use the old cups from the kitchen for mixing paint in the craft workshop. If we do then we should not be surprised when a client does the same thing with our brand new best china.

- If you are introducing an object to a person for the first time, teach them exactly what it is for and how to use it. Do not make jokes about it or do anything that might confuse the person about the use of the object.

- If a person misuses an object, do not be impatient with them. Avoid saying things like "use that properly"; as far as the person is concerned they may already believe that they are using it properly.

- Teach the correct use by showing the person how to use the object, give this correct use a name. When you want the person to use the object correctly, help them understand by using the name of the correct use, eg when teaching a person to use a broom for sweeping, call the activity 'sweeping'. In future, when you ask the person to use a broom, always add that you want them to use it for sweeping.

- Do not indulge in horseplay that demonstrates the wrong use of an object. Using a cup to throw water over a colleague on a hot summer day in the garden is not just silly, it may also lead to a client throwing the (possibly hot) contents of a cup over someone in the future.

- If you are working with someone who cannot understand the real purpose of an object they misuse then try to reduce the amount of contact they can have with that object. The amount of contact varies with the danger created by the way the object is misused. A person who thinks that drinking glasses are for spinning is at risk of cutting themselves if the glass breaks. You must accept responsibility for supervising their use of glasses or for making sure that they have a safer alternative available.

- Some forms of misusing objects seem unimportant until the person is out in open society where their behaviour may make them look extremely odd to other people. The best place to teach the person not to misuse the object is within their own home, where you can repeat the teaching in a relaxed environment. DO NOT leave such teaching until the behaviour becomes a problem; both you and the client will be more tense, and less able to deal with the matter in a relaxed way.

Notes

TASK

If you were able to identify someone you work with as being a person who uses objects without awareness of their real use, describe their behaviour on Worksheet 17. Think through the above points and decide which ones may be of some help in helping the person to handle those objects more appropriately. Describe how you would approach changing their behaviour.

Your plan will be specific to one client only, as it would not necessarily be appropriate for anybody else who has a similar difficulty. Consider how you might have to adapt this approach to help other clients.

Remember that you should not try to implement your plan without the agreement of your line manager and the rest of the staff team.

WORKING WITH THE TRIAD

Description of present behaviour

_____

_____

_____

_____

_____

_____

_____

_____

_____

_____

_____

_____

Plan for helping change that behaviour

_____

_____

_____

_____

_____

_____

_____

_____

_____

_____

_____

_____

IMPAIRMENT OF IMAGINATION AND SOCIAL UNDERSTANDING

Inflexibility in applying written and unwritten social rules and inflexibility of thought

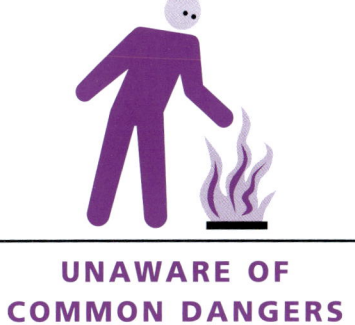

UNAWARE OF COMMON DANGERS

We are used to the idea that many people with learning disabilities are unaware of common dangers because of their lack of understanding. Where people with a learning disability also have autism, we need to be aware of the extra difficulty created for them.

Some people with autism are at greater risk because of the impairment of their imagination and social understanding. One effect of this impairment can be that the person is inflexible in their thinking. Even if there is only a mild degree of learning disability or no learning disability at all, the following kind of problems can occur.

Someone who has been taught never to run across the road may still not run when they misjudge a crossing and see a car heading for them. The person who has been taught never to put their hand on a cooker when the electric rings are red may think that the red colour is the danger and burn themselves on rings that are dark but still hot enough to burn.

Inflexibility of thought also puts the person at risk when they do what they have been taught to, without realising that the situation calls for a 'bending' of the normal rules, eg the person who has been taught always to put their dressing gown and slippers on before leaving their bedroom: in the case of fire in the building they are likely to stop to find these and to put them on, instead of getting out as fast as they can.

 EXERCISE

Can you identify inflexibility of thought as being a problem for any of the people you work with? This may be a display of anxiety when something is in the 'wrong' place; a belief that a trip out will necessarily include visits to certain places; a particular way of leaving or entering the building; a fear of something that was a problem just once, possibly a long time ago. Ask your line manager to help you if you find this exercise difficult. Do any of the examples you can identify mean that the person could be at risk?

Notes
....

REMEMBER

A person who has done what they were taught to do, rather than react in a flexible way to avoid danger, will be confused if you criticise them. Accept your responsibility for supervising the person more closely.

Never leave it to the people you are caring for to adapt their behaviour because there is a risk of danger. They may be incapable of doing so.

WAYS OF HELPING

- Be aware of situations where following the normal 'rules' could create danger. Do not expect your clients to understand this for themselves. Take responsibility for guiding them out of the danger.

- Avoid giving clients poor quality instructions/training that increase the possibility of them being exposed to risk or danger, eg showing someone that they can use a knife to remove bread that has become stuck in the toaster is very poor training. They may attempt to do this without remembering to switch the toaster off or may not realise which socket the toaster is plugged into in the first place.

- People with autism are known to have repetitive behaviours. They must complete these before they can do anything else. Do not expect them to hurry up, to stop or to change their ritual just because there is a risk of danger present. Someone who always taps their hand six times on the light switch before they can leave the room, will continue to do so, even when the switch is broken and live wires are exposed.

- Some people with autism have a strong need for things to be just where they think they should be. Someone who is troubled by a curtain partly coming off the rail may try to reach up to put it right. To reach the curtain rail they may climb on chairs, or onto the window ledge, and be at risk of falling. Make sure that such things are dealt with promptly by staff to reduce the risk to the client(s) concerned.

- Anxiety about something can rob the person of their ability to think about other important things going on around them, eg the person who is frightened of dogs may be so alarmed at seeing a dog in the distance that they rush across the road without thinking of the road drill they have been taught. We need to know which people have anxieties that might lead to them putting themselves at risk. When they become anxious it is our responsibility to provide closer supervision and support.

TASK

If you have a person who displays a lack of awareness of common dangers amongst the clients you are working with, use Worksheet 18 to describe the problem they present. Think through the points above and describe the steps you should take to try and reduce the risk to the person as much as is possible.

Your plan will be specific to one client only, as it would not necessarily be appropriate for anybody else who has a similar difficulty. Consider how you might have to adapt this approach to help other clients.

Remember that you should not try to implement your plan without the agreement of your line manager and the rest of the staff team.

Notes

....

WORKING WITH THE TRIAD

Description of present behaviour

_____

_____

_____

_____

_____

_____

_____

_____

_____

_____

_____

_____

_____

Plan for helping change that behaviour

_____

_____

_____

_____

_____

_____

_____

_____

_____

_____

_____

_____

IMPAIRMENT OF IMAGINATION AND SOCIAL UNDERSTANDING

Difficulty in understanding that others may have a different view

Inflexibility of thought

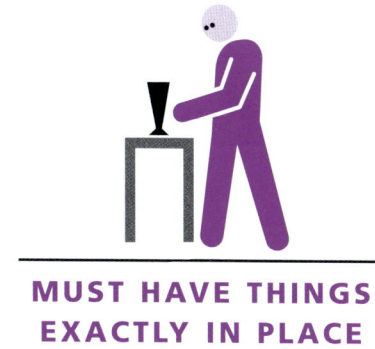

MUST HAVE THINGS EXACTLY IN PLACE

Some people with autism can be very rigid in their understanding of where things should be. Walking into a room and noticing that something is in the 'wrong' place, they have a strong need to put the object where they believe it should be.

This behaviour is due to the inflexibility of thought that arises from the impairment of imagination and social understanding. Once the person has their own view of where objects should be they feel ill at ease if any of them are moved. They may feel equally ill at ease if something new is added to the room.

Just like you, people with autism do not like feeling ill at ease and they are motivated to put things 'right', so that they can relax.

The impairment of imagination and social understanding also makes it difficult for people with autism to appreciate that others may have a different point of view to their own. No matter how you try to explain the reasons for an object having to be moved, the person with autism may find it difficult to understand. The idea that the majority of people like the object in its new position and wish it to stay there, is equally hard for them to understand.

Sometimes the problems raised by this behaviour seem to be impossible to solve. Someone who is compelled to put the kitchen utensils in the drawer will keep on putting them away, even when someone else is using them to cook a meal.

Occasionally the behaviour extends to adjusting other people's clothes whilst they are wearing them. Someone who believes that jackets must be done up may become very distressed when they meet someone with an unbuttoned jacket, and continually try to do it up for them.

EXERCISE

Observe the people you are caring for and identify any behaviour that seems to fit the description of 'must have things exactly in place' or fits the examples of behaviour that are given above. What happens when they cannot put things how they want them to be? Do they usually achieve their objective of putting it 'right' at some point in the day?

REMEMBER

This behaviour is not always a problem. A mild case is called tidiness and is seen as appropriate behaviour. In the person's own room it may be seen as 'self-determination'. The behaviour only becomes a problem in extreme cases. Insistence on having things exactly in place, where it disrupts normal everyday living may be seen as a repetitive behaviour or ritual. This aspect of the person with autism is dealt with in Section 4.

WAYS OF HELPING

- When you are introducing people to a new environment try to get things as right as possible before they move in. Adding a fire extinguisher, a new wall 'phone or a house plant can cause anxiety for people who do not think these things should be there. They are quite likely to keep removing them.

- Do not get locked into foolish battles of will with the person. If they want things just so in their own room accept that as their right. If they want things just so in a lounge used by everyone, ask yourself if the other clients mind. If they don't mind ask yourself why you do, before you decide that you must change the behaviour of the person.

- Remember that the person might be at risk if they attempt to climb up to straighten lamp shades, or re-hook a curtain. Deal with such things yourself as soon as you see them. If it is something you cannot deal with, report the matter under your Health and Safety procedures as it does affect the safety of the client.

- Be ready to distract a person who may try to readjust the clothing of other people. It is not reasonable to expect other clients to accept this behaviour. Staff should not accept it happening to them either, and doing so is a poor example to set. Members of the public will not like having their clothing tucked in, buttoned up, or straightened for them.

- Work with all other staff to keep a record of exactly when this behaviour occurs. Note what was happening for that client immediately before they began it. This behaviour is often linked to anxiety, the person using it to lessen feelings of anxiety which may have initially been caused by something quite different. We need to know what might have caused that anxiety; if we can prevent it in future this problem behaviour might not appear so often.

- In addition to trying to identify specific reasons why the person may become anxious, we also need to reduce their general level of anxiety. A person who feels in control of their lives will have less need to control exactly where furniture and ornaments are put.

Notes

TASK

If you were able to identify this behaviour in one of the people you work with, use Worksheet 19 to describe their behaviour. Read through the general points above and write a suggestion of how you might work with the person to help them become less concerned about the things they are trying to control.

Your plan will be specific to one client only, as it would not necessarily be appropriate for anybody else who has a similar difficulty. Consider how you might have to adapt this approach to help other clients.

Remember that you should not try to implement your plan without the agreement of your line manager and the rest of the staff team.

WORKING WITH THE TRIAD

Description of present behaviour

_____

_____

_____

_____

_____

_____

_____

_____

_____

_____

_____

_____

Plan for helping change that behaviour

_____

_____

_____

_____

_____

_____

_____

_____

_____

_____

_____

_____

IMPAIRMENT OF IMAGINATION AND SOCIAL UNDERSTANDING

A minority of people with autism display talents or abilities far greater than their general level of development would suggest. This is not restricted to people with autism, but may also be seen in others with a learning disability. Often the ability is in music or art. People with autism who display special talents often do so in the areas of memory and mental arithmetic.

Not all these special abilities are particularly useful though. Being exceptionally skilled at dismantling (but not reassembling) electronic equipment; remembering the names and birth dates of all the people you have ever been introduced to; memorising the British Rail timetable, to name a few examples, might be regarded as less than useful.

It may be that these special abilities develop in some people with autism because of the inflexibility of thought and the obsessions that many of them have. For instance, the ability to spend all one's free hours obsessively operating a computer to the exclusion of social and other activities is likely to help some individuals become very good at computer programming.

Although you may not be working with someone with autism whose special abilities could be thought of as a socially acceptable talent or gift, can you recognise any area of unusually high ability amongst the clients you know?

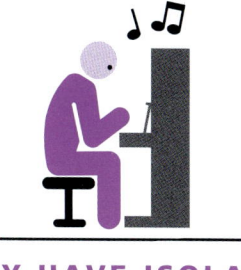

MAY HAVE ISOLATED AREA OF ABILITY

REPETITIVE BEHAVIOURS

INTRODUCTION

You may have noticed that some of the people you are working with have patterns of behaviour (sometimes odd or bizarre) that they repeat again and again. You may see the behaviour repeated many times per day or just a few times each week. These repeated behaviours may be simple ones such as twiddling with objects or simple bodily movements, but some may be very complex behaviours which may be described as ritualistic, such as insisting on getting dressed or undressed in exactly the same way every time. These repetitive or ritualistic behaviours can assume very great importance to the person displaying them, who might become very distressed if they are interfered with.

When he first identified autism in 1943, the psychiatrist Leo Kanner described 'the repetitive and stereotyped' play activities that he had noticed amongst the children he was describing. In 1945, working quite separately to Kanner, an Austrian, Hans Asperger, who was studying a similar group of children, described the 'rituals and obsessions' displayed by them.

In this section you will look at some examples of repetitive or ritualistic behaviour and follow through some ideas about why it occurs. Most importantly you will look at ways in which you can help people whose behaviour is often repetitive or ritualistic.

Do not worry about fine distinctions between the terms repetitive and ritualistic. For the purposes of this section, repetitive will generally refer to the simple behaviours, ritual or ritualistic will generally refer to the more complex behaviours and routines. However a repetitive behaviour might be described as a ritual for simplicity.

There is a lot of information for you to work through in this section. Do not rush through it or you will find it difficult to understand all the detail. Understanding repetitive behaviour is important in your work with people with autism – take time to learn about it.

You will be familiar with the term 'Active but Odd', which is used to describe behaviour relating to the impairment of social relating skills. You will remember that the typical behaviour types were:

1 Aloof   **2** Passive   **3** Active but Odd.

When thinking about repetitive behaviour it is important to remember that behaviour that looks odd does not automatically place the person in the Active but Odd group. Repetitive behaviour, which may certainly look odd, is seen in all three groups. The term 'Active but Odd' applies to social relating behaviour.

TASK

Spend the next few days you are at work watching the clients you work with to see if you can identify any repetitive behaviours that individuals may be displaying. Use Worksheet 20 to record your observations. Discuss your findings with your study supervisor before going on to work on the rest of the section.

WORKSHEET
20

REPETITIVE BEHAVIOURS

OBSERVATION OF REPETITIVE BEHAVIOUR

Description of present behaviour

CASE STUDY: OLIVER

You will now begin following the case study of Oliver (not his real name), which has been used to help you understand the key points in this section. You will find more episodes of the case study as you go through this section. Read the case study material through at least twice to make sure you have taken notice of all the points raised.

OLIVER

Oliver is a 24-year-old man with autism and with associated learning disability. Oliver has no speech but clearly understands familiar words and sentences. Apart from the signs for 'toilets' and 'please' Oliver has no means of communicating with other people except through his behaviour. As a young child Oliver frequently became distressed. Sometimes this led to bouts of screaming. At other times he would bite the back of his hands, and hit out at his parents.

Although he made little progress at his special school, Oliver seemed to enjoy his life; his school reports show a rapid calming down by the age 10. Socially passive in his behaviour Oliver made few demands on his teachers and classmates but usually seemed to be happy enough to go along with what was happening around him. Home life was not so peaceful during these years. Oliver's parents remember that they often wondered if he would be happier in a residential school.

Oliver's parents reported that he had a number of repetitive behaviours during his childhood. Bending down to touch each step every time he went up stairs lasted until he was eight years old; repeatedly turning light switches on and off lasted for two years; waving his vest over his head exactly eight times before putting it on happened every day between the ages of 12 to 15 years. Any attempt to stop Oliver performing these rituals led to him becoming very distressed.

On leaving school Oliver attended an adult day centre. On the first day there he began a new ritual: many times each day he dropped to a sitting position on the floor and rapidly removed both his shoes and his socks; he then sat tapping his shoes on the floor. Oliver had no objection to members of staff putting his shoes and socks on again for him, in fact he rather seemed to enjoy the process.

Oliver's parents tried different kinds of shoes, including tightly buckled sandals. Oliver became very skilled at removing all forms of footwear in a matter of moments. For a few months, this ritual led to him being placed in the special care unit of the day centre because it did not

Notes
....

matter if he walked about in bare feet in there. Consequently Oliver was excluded from many of the centre's activities, particularly those going on in the local community.

It was eventually decided that it was not in Oliver's best interests to remain in the special care unit and he was brought back into the main day centre where the process of trying to change his behaviour was begun.

Why do repetitive behaviours occur?

Kanner described children with autism as having a 'desire for sameness'. Observing the children he noticed that they often tried to make the same thing happen today as happened at that time yesterday. Certainly some of the behaviours we call rituals may start in that way.

Of course people with autism do not become repetitive about everything they have experienced. We also know that rituals often seem to appear from nowhere and do not always seem to be learnt from previous experience.

As Oliver's parents found, rituals seem to keep on appearing in the life of some people with autism. Nobody seems able to say why a particular behaviour or action becomes a ritual, or how long it will last, or why it goes away.

Often when a ritual does disappear it is almost immediately replaced by a new one. It is as though some people with autism need to have rituals in their lives. If we are to help them we need to try and work out why that may be.

People like Oliver are not the only ones to have rituals. All human beings are repetitive to some extent. Do you tap your fingers sometimes? Twiddle your hair? Bite your nails? Always watch the same soap opera? Always walk the dog at the same time? Always go to the pub/restaurant/cinema/etc. on Saturday night?

 EXERCISE

Think through your own behaviour. Do you have any repetitive behaviours that could be described as a ritual? Think particularly about behaviours and actions that you carry out when you are feeling stressed or worried.

Complete the personal rituals exercise on the next page.

Consider why you have rituals.

REPETITIVE BEHAVIOURS   EXERCISE

PERSONAL RITUALS EXERCISE

Repetitive behaviours and rituals ease us through our lives and play a positive role in reassuring us and helping us to mark special occasions. Think about the considerable ritual involved in such occasions as religious ceremonies, weddings and deaths, for instance.

To help you to understand the role that rituals play in our lives, and the role that they could play in the lives of people with autism, please complete the following exercise.

1. **List some of your morning (getting up) rituals**
   Some examples of morning rituals may include:

   Setting the alarm early enough so that you can press the snooze alarm twice before getting up; always washing your hair first when you have a shower; listening to a particular radio programme; must have that cup of coffee first; reading a particular newspaper.

2. **List your night-time rituals**
   For example, what do you always do when preparing to retire?

REPETITIVE BEHAVIOURS   EXERCISE

3. List some of your rituals of transition (starting a new activity)

For example, what do you always do when you arrive at work?

For example, what do you always do when you arrive home?

4. List some of your weekly rituals

For example, how do you like to spend Sunday morning (if you are not working)?

REPETITIVE BEHAVIOURS

EXERCISE

Which regular weekly rituals do you have (TV programmes you always watch; sports that you always watch or play, people or places you always visit, etc?)

5. **List some of your rituals of celebration and comfort**

For example, how do you like to celebrate when something good happens (tell someone, go out for dinner, have a drink, buy something special)?

For example, how do you comfort yourself when something unpleasant happens? How do you make yourself feel better?

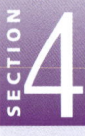
REPETITIVE BEHAVIOURS   EXERCISE

6. List some special occasion and holiday rituals

For example, what has to happen in order for you to enjoy your birthday?

For example, what foods have to be on the table at which holidays (eg Christmas)?

For example, what do you have to do during particular holidays (eg visit relatives)?

REPETITIVE BEHAVIOURS   EXERCISE

7. What are some of the other rituals in your life?
For example, there are rituals in relationships – you always wash the dishes whilst your partner dries.

_____

_____

_____

_____

_____

8. List any rituals which hinder you
For example, are you unable to leave the house unless you have checked all the windows and doors? Do you always have to make a detour around ladders to avoid walking under them?

_____

_____

_____

_____

_____

9. The balance between positive and negative rituals
Do the majority of your rituals and repetitive behaviours help you in your life or do they hinder you?

Do you value your rituals and repetitive behaviours?

How would you feel if some all-powerful authority tried to deny you your rituals and repetitive behaviours?

_____

_____

_____

_____

_____

Now go on to complete Worksheet 21 on the following page.

REPETITIVE BEHAVIOURS

POSITIVE RITUALS

Think about, and write a short discussion on, how rituals might be used positively in the lives of the people we support.

_____

_____

_____

_____

_____

_____

_____

_____

_____

_____

_____

_____

_____

_____

_____

_____

_____

_____

_____

_____

_____

_____

_____

_____

THE LINK BETWEEN RITUALS AND STRESS

Stress comes in many forms. In a physical sense we are used to the idea that too much weight on a bridge will strain the structure, causing it to weaken or collapse.

In terms of our mental wellbeing, stress is somewhat harder to define. Things that worry us or cause us to feel insecure certainly cause us stress. In extreme circumstances, if we have too much worry or feel too insecure, we can suffer a mental collapse – commonly known as a 'nervous breakdown'.

All of us have some stress in our lives, different levels at different times and situations. The secret of a happy life is not to have no stress at all but to avoid too much stress at any one time. Indeed stress can be a help to us – it is an effective motivator, for instance.

When we are over-stressed we feel physically uncomfortable. This is because our bodies react to stress in a particular way. When we become anxious or worried, our body chemistry changes. Adrenalin is automatically added to our blood and has the effect of quickly turning some of our fat into sugar, thus providing us with extra energy. Our throats can dry up; we may feel 'butterflies' in our stomachs; our blood pressure rises slightly and we begin to breathe faster, pulling more oxygen into our bodies. All this is to prepare us for 'fight or flight', the body assuming that stress equals danger and getting itself ready to either fight that danger or to run away from it.

However, most of the stress we experience is not caused by things that we need to run away from or fight. Despite this we will have extra energy in our bodies making us want to be more active. If we are in a social situation we usually cannot get up and run around, so we twiddle, tap or fidget instead, as they are about the only socially acceptable things we can do in the circumstances.

People with autism often do not have the same concern about what is socially acceptable behaviour. When they feel stressed they have the same reaction as the rest of us but are more inclined to burn off the energy they feel inside by jumping up, moving around, tapping windows, flicking light switches, etc.

Behaviour which happens frequently, apparently without good reason or purpose, is often called ritualistic. Perhaps it is a guide to how much stress the person with autism is feeling and an increase in such behaviour indicates increased stress.

Notes

Notes

....

WHY SHOULD PEOPLE WITH AUTISM SUFFER FROM STRESS?

People with autism have the Triad of Impairments and often have learning disabilities as well. Consider how would you feel if:

1. You had problems in understanding and interacting with the people around you. Perhaps you want to relate to others but don't know how to.

2. You had problems communicating with and understanding the rest of the human race. Perhaps you could recognise some of the words people use but not the tone of voice, facial expressions, and body language that give the words their meaning.

3. You had problems in understanding how other people see things and had difficulty in understanding how the written laws and social customs that govern life are changed, depending on the circumstances at the time.

And if, on top of all this, you were constantly given instructions and explanations which you could not understand, by people who behaved towards you as though you *do* understand and are choosing not to comply.

RESPONSE TO STRESS

 EXERCISE

Imagine yourself in the situation described below. Explain how you would most likely be feeling and what you would do in such a situation.

You are lost in the centre of what is obviously a crowded foreign city. All the street signs are written in a script which you cannot read and you are surrounded by a large crowd of people, all of whom are of a different race and who are speaking a language you do not understand. The people seem to be trying to tell you something important and they are impatient. Some begin to shout and move towards you. You feel the urgency of the situation and wonder what is going to happen next; you begin to fear for your safety.

RESPONSE TO STRESS   EXERCISE

How would you be feeling – emotionally and physically?

How would you be likely to respond? – consider your options.

Can you think of any ritual/s which may help?

THE TRIAD OF IMPAIRMENTS AS A CAUSE OF STRESS

"The changes people make in terms of touch, sound, movement, and emotion, make life a sensory hell from which to run and hide, or tirelessly try to control…"

"…the only warmth is in the colours, patterns, sounds, smells, and textures of things which stay the same long enough to be seen as trustworthy…"

"…the constant change of the people world rocks a concrete sense of perfection and predictability…"

Extracts from **Nobody Nowhere** *by Donna Williams, published by Doubleday 1992*

An able woman with autism, Donna Williams gives us a chance to read how someone with this condition feels about the life they have led.

At a meeting in London, an American woman with autism, Temple Grandin, who has also written about her life, made the following comment:

"…every day of my life, coping with everyday things causes me as much stress as you might feel on the day you took your final exams to qualify for your future career…"

CASE STUDY:

OLIVER (continued)

The attempt to help Oliver started with an assessment of his repetitive behaviour. Staff were asked to record every occasion when Oliver removed his shoes and socks. After one month all the record sheets were carefully checked. The first thing that was noticed was that Oliver did not remove his shoes and socks 'all the time' as people had been saying. He actually removed them 244 times during that month. Now the centre had a figure that it could use as a check to see if the behaviour became more frequent or less frequent as time went on.

Staff were asked to continue their observation for another month, this time recording what was happening when Oliver removed his shoes and socks. When these records were checked it was discovered that Oliver usually took his shoes and socks off when somebody asked him to do something. This was not always true. When asked to go for his drink at break time, his meal at lunch time, or to get his coat on to go home, Oliver never took his shoes and socks off.

KNOWING WHAT COMES NEXT

People with autism often have difficulty in understanding what is happening around them. How do you feel when you do not know what is happening, or what is going to happen next, or when nobody tells you what is going on?

Think about a situation you have experienced where you did not know what was going to happen next, perhaps your first day in a new job or an interview for a job you really wanted, after which you were sent away with no idea how well you had done, to wait for a letter.

When we cannot predict, or guess what might happen next, most of us feel a bit insecure. Depending on the circumstances we might actually feel frightened. Either way, not knowing what is going to happen next causes people to feel stress, because if they do not know what is coming next they cannot be sure they will be able to cope with it, so:

- the body gets itself ready for flight or fight again

- the changes in body chemistry lead to repetitive behaviour.

CASE STUDY:

OLIVER (continued)

Finding that Oliver never took his shoes and socks off before meal breaks or before going home made staff at the centre scratch their heads for a while. What did this mean? Perhaps Oliver was just behaving better when he liked something. The staff team felt happy with this idea, adding that Oliver was a bit lazy and probably just took his shoes off to try and avoid work.

As that explanation did not help anybody decide what to do to change Oliver's behaviour, staff were asked to think about the following ideas.

Oliver understood exactly what was happening when he was asked to go for a drink or a meal. He also understood exactly what was meant by instructions to get ready to go home at the end of the day. Because he

Notes
....

understood these things he did not feel any anxiety about them so was not stressed.

Because of his autism, Oliver found it hard to understand other kinds of instruction such as "let's do self-care now" or "let's go for a walk into town". Because he did not understand quite what was expected of him or exactly what was going to happen next, he began to experience anxiety which caused the stress which was causing the ritual of taking his shoes and socks off. The behaviour was simply Oliver's stress release behaviour, such as we may tap our fingers or twiddle with our hair.

This is more than a guess – Oliver's history is a clue to why these ideas might be correct. He did not have repetitive behaviour at school, where he would have had a very structured, easy-to-understand timetable. His parents report long complicated rituals as being a continual part of his home life. Family homes are rarely highly organised and structured places. They are full of sudden events, unusual treats and surprises for the children; relaxed days when nobody bothers with activities, etc. Home life would have been harder for Oliver to understand and to feel secure within.

RITUALS MAKE PEOPLE FEEL BETTER

When people carry out a ritual because they are feeling stressed, the behaviour comforts them. This is for two reasons:

1. By doing something, they are using up the energy released by their bodies in response to the stress.

2. A ritual is something the person does so often that it is familiar to them. As it is familiar it feels safe, the opposite to whatever is worrying them. People feel in control of their own rituals and are comforted by them.

So, repetitive behaviour helps people to cope with stressful situations.

Go back to the section which asked you to identify your own rituals. If you are a finger or foot tapper when you are anxious, how does tapping your fingers help? If you are not sure how to reply, think how you feel when you want to tap your fingers (or whatever) but someone else tells you to stop it.

CASE STUDY:

OLIVER (continued)

Working with the idea that Oliver's repetitive behaviour was a response to anxiety and stress, and that his anxiety and stress were caused by him not understanding what was happening around him, the staff at the day centre drew up new programmes for Oliver to follow.

The programmes were structured, each moment of each day being planned so that staff could more easily offer Oliver the certainty of what came next in his activities.

Every activity session was followed by a break for a drink, a meal or a favoured activity so that even if Oliver was uncertain about an activity session, he could be comforted by knowing that something he did understand came next.

In the first month of the new programmes, Oliver took his shoes and socks off 301 times, an increase that led some staff to doubt the new programmes. Staff were asked to give the programmes more time, as the programmes were new to Oliver and he could be expected to feel more anxiety until he got used to them.

In the second month Oliver took his shoes and socks off 260 times;

the third month, 148 times;

the fourth month, 57 times;

the fifth month, 43 times;

the sixth month, 11 times.

REMEMBER

The taking his shoes and socks off ritual was caused by Oliver feeling stressed because he could not understand that was happening now and what was coming next. As he was used to his own ritual, doing it comforted him. The ritual also had a second effect, also comforting to Oliver: it made it possible for Oliver to become quite certain of what came next – what always happened when he took his shoes and socks off?

Answer – staff always put them back on for him.

Notes

Notes
....

HELPING PEOPLE WITH REPETITIVE BEHAVIOUR

1. Do not simply decide to discourage or try to stop the repetitive behaviour. It may be the only way the person has to cope with feelings of stress and to comfort him/herself when feeling anxious. If you stop such a behaviour, another one is likely to appear soon afterwards as the person still needs some way of coping with anxiety and stress.

2. Accept that the person is very likely to have anxiety and stress in their life, even if it is not obvious to you why that should be.

3. Reach agreement with the staff team about exactly what the behaviour is.

4. Agree a period of observation and record:

   a) how many times the behaviour occurs;

   b) the time that it occurs;

   c) what was happening just before the behaviour began.

5. Draw all observations together and work out:

   a) how many times the behaviour is occurring each day or week;

   b) if it occurs at some times and not others;

   c) if there is any obvious problem raising the person's anxiety just before their behaviour starts.

6. If the observations are inconclusive, continue them for a longer period.

7. If a pattern is found that suggests that the behaviour is linked to something stressful in the person's life, plan how that stress can be reduced, either by changing the event or by helping the person understand it more clearly.

8. If no clear pattern is found, change observations to determine:

   a) if the person can communicate their own needs effectively;

   b) if the person finds crowded or noisy rooms/activities stressful;

   c) if the person really understands the language used by carers/trainers;

   d) if the person understands the structure of their day (they should know and understand what is coming next and what is required of them).

9. Depending on your findings provide either:

    a) communication training;

    b) reduce noise levels/number of people in the vicinity;

    c) check the person's vocabulary to determine exactly what words they fully understand. Do not use words they cannot understand, teach the new words they need or teach signs, or provide pictures or symbols;

    d) structure the person's day; give them a personal timetable and use pictures if words are not understood.

10. Make sure that timetables and structures allow for each activity to end in an easily-understood activity, such as a break or meal time. Keep to the structure you have set up to help the person; if you let it break down you will cause anxiety and stress.

Notes

WORKSHEET 22

OVERCOMING PROBLEM BEHAVIOUR

Use the guidelines on the previous page to observe and analyse the behaviour, and devise a strategy which will help overcome the problems which the behaviour causes.

Description of present behaviour:
(You should have a particular client in mind, though it is not necessary to name him/her here)

_____

_____

_____

_____

_____

_____

_____

_____

_____

_____

Observations

_____

_____

_____

_____

_____

_____

_____

_____

_____

_____

_____

_____

Continue on next page

WORKSHEET

Plan for helping to overcome the problems it causes

INTRODUCTION

In this section you will be looking at why we need adhere to consistent work practices in our work with people who have autistic spectrum disorders.

One of the most common problems raised by teams of care staff is their own understanding that they are not consistent in their work, and that clients suffer because of this.

People with autism are considerably disadvantaged by the inconsistent behaviour of the people who look after them. In most care settings this is not so important because most people are reassured by common social gestures such as a smile, a pat on the shoulder, a hug, etc. These gestures show that they are cared for and provide some peace of mind. However the majority of people with autism are not sure what these gestures mean and so are not comforted by them. They are dependent on familiar patterns of activity and behaviour for their reassurance and peace of mind, which is why it is so important that we are consistent in our behaviour and in the way we present activities.

In the last section on repetitive behaviours, you saw quotes from Donna Williams' book *Nobody Nowhere*, in which she describes her life as a person with autism. They are worth repeating here:

"…the spontaneity and constant change of the people world rocks a concrete sense of perfection and predictability…"

"…the changes people make in terms of touch, sound, movement and emotion make life a sensory hell from which to run and hide, or tirelessly try to control…"

Think about the way your mood affects your behaviour, how you behave when you feel in good spirits against how you behave when you are tired and grumpy.

Donna Williams is talking about you… and the rest of us.

We take for granted that people's behaviour changes depending on their mood. We can empathise – we can imagine what it is like to be another person. We understand. People with autistic spectrum disorders do not empathise and they cannot learn to do so. They remain mystified though they may learn to cope – to a degree.

CREATING AND MAINTAINING CONSISTENT WORK PRACTICES

The two major areas of the client's life over which we have some control are:

1. the environment

2. ourselves and our colleagues.

By carefully monitoring and controlling these we may begin to provide a framework of consistent factors which will provide reassuring predictability for the clients.

1. The environment

We can expect people who have variously been described as 'seeking to maintain sameness' (Leo Kanner), 'showing resistance to change' (Hans Asperger) and having 'inflexibility of thought' (Lorna Wing) to prefer to live in physical surroundings that stay the same.

To quote Donna Williams again:

"…the only warmth is in the colours, patterns, sounds, textures, and smells of things that stay the same long enough to be considered trustworthy…"

Keeping the housing and the workshops that we run as 'trustworthy' environments sounds simple enough, but in reality it is quite difficult. Flooring materials wear out, furniture becomes shabby, walls become dirty and need redecorating. Sometimes we may need to alter the building itself.

Fortunately, the majority of people with autism can cope with change. What they seem to find very difficult is change that they are not expecting, that which takes them by surprise. Having once experienced the shock of unexpected change they seem to find it very difficult to build up their trust again. Their anxiety rather suggests that once something has been shown to change without warning, they believe that it can do so again at any time.

Writing in the National Autistic Society's magazine *Communication* some years ago, the mother of a boy with autism recalled how her husband had taken a day off work to redecorate their son's bedroom. When he came home from school and was taken by a proud father to see his new room the child was violently distressed by the change, refused to go into the room, and has not done so since.

Notes

Notes
....

2. The people

It is much harder to achieve consistent, predictable patterns of behaviour from people. Modern life and care practice encourages us to be informal and relaxed in our work, turning up for work in various frames of mind and behaving in ways limited only by colleagues. We expect our colleagues to make allowances for us if we are feeling tired and irritable after a late night, are hung over, are upset by difficulties in a relationship, etc.

What we are inclined to forget is that our workplace is usually other people's homes (the people we care for) and that it is not our colleagues whom we should defer to, but the clients.

People with autism can usually cope with our appearance changing: hair gets cut, beards grow and vanish, skirts are replaced by jeans; earrings are worn, or not; glasses are replaced by contact lenses, etc. In many cases people with autism hardly seem to notice, though some will be intensely interested by these details.

What they do seem to notice and can be greatly affected by, are our moods, our tone of voice, the volume of our speech. Often we seem to be known to the client in terms of our temperament.

Of course it is not just people with autism who are affected, we all know of people who use changes of mood – moving from good humour to displays of temper, suddenly and without warning – as a means of exercising power over others. Many of us will know what it is like to be subject to the whims of a powerful personality who can make us feel upset or inadequate. Many people use the power of their behaviour to exercise control over others by keeping people 'off balance' and unsure how to respond. Their power comes from causing feelings of insecurity in others which disempowers or disables them.

If this abuse of power can have such a disabling effect on us, think how easy it would be to exercise such power over people who are socially disabled. It can and often is done completely unconsciously unless we become very aware of our behaviour and its powerful effects on others.

It would not be reasonable or realistic to expect members of a staff team all to behave in exactly the same way. Our personalities are so different that it would be impossible, even if we tried. Having different personalities in a staff group also enriches the experience of people with autism, widening their experience and opportunities to relate to different people.

People with autism do not need us to all behave in the same way, like robots. What would greatly help them, and ourselves in our dealings with them, would be for each one of us to behave in a consistent, predictable way every day. To do this we have to put our own feelings and needs aside and consider those of the clients.

Notes

> ### ▶ EXERCISE
>
> List the different moods that you know you have, and put the one that describes how you are most of the time at the top of the list.
>
> _____
>
> _____
>
> _____
>
> _____
>
> _____
>
> Now list the moods that are likely to make you seem different today as far as the clients are concerned.
>
> _____
>
> _____
>
> _____
>
> _____
>
> Lastly, list those moods that you find hardest to control when you are at work.
>
> _____
>
> _____
>
> _____
>
> _____
>
> _____

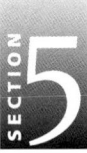

Notes

You must take responsibility for managing your behaviour. If you are normally a relaxed person who is tolerant of clients' behaviours, then do not bring a rare bad temper to work and change the way you relate to the clients. They will be totally confused by the change in your behaviour. You may make them anxious or even lose their confidence and trust in you.

Leave your unusual moods, especially the ones you find hard to control, outside of the workplace. You would understand people being confused if you turned up in clown's costume, your face heavily made up. Remember that behaving like a clown would be even more confusing for people with autism because they have an impairment of social understanding and cannot interpret your behaviour.

Managing planned change

When we know that something in the environment is going to change, we must make it as stress-free as possible for the people with autism who are going to be involved in that change. Points to remember are:

- Always tell people well in advance, even if it means they will become anxious and demand a lot of reassurance from you. That is the point of telling them, so that they can ask for reassurance if they need it, and get it.

- Describe the limits of the change, eg "We are painting the corridor outside your room but we are not painting inside your room". Don't wait for the person to ask, tell them as part of your management of the change.

- Where possible let clients make some decisions about the change. Where a person is at least partly in control of changes, they do not seem to be so anxious about them.

- If the person cannot understand the language, signs or pictograms that you could use to keep them informed of changes, try to let them see at least the start of the work. Never bring them into familiar surroundings that have changed whilst they were absent.

- Where a person becomes anxious about change, do not brush their anxiety aside and wait for them to get used to it. Offer the person support. If necessary re-train them to understand and use that part of the environment that has changed. Set your re-training at the same level of support the person would need if they were newly arrived clients.

- Be consistent in your approach to clients. If you realise that you have acted differently from normal, offer the person reassurance and support as soon as you have your mood under control.

- Keep your voice tone and volume under control so that you do not sound different from day to day.

- Ensure that staff handover procedures are followed and used effectively. Staff can only achieve a consistent approach to clients if they pool their knowledge of how the person is today and what is known to be happening in their lives.

- Remember that trips out for the clients are just that, for the clients. Keep your mood and behaviour in your normal range, despite your feelings about it.

- Know, and at all times be honest with yourself about how you are behaving. Remember that your behaviour is visible for all to see. You are not fooling anybody, especially those who depend on you.

INDIVIDUAL PROGRAMME PLANS AND TIMETABLES

You will probably have already seen the individual programme plans (IPPs) for the clients and, perhaps, have contributed to a meeting called to review that programme.

If they are to be effective, they must at least ensure two things:

1 That the person's abilities and needs have been identified, and a plan for increasing their abilities and meeting their needs has been designed.

2 That all staff who come into contact with that person have written guidelines for exactly what approach they should take with that person in any important respect.

Even when there is a properly constructed IPP, there is no guarantee of a consistent approach. If staff do not read the guidelines or follow them conscientiously, then all the work which went into the planning is sabotaged and the IPP is useless.

Timetables exist to present the planned structure of the day/week/month to both staff and clients. Timetables can be written for each individual as an extension of their IPP, or can be written for groups of people who are coming together to share an activity.

Notes

Individual timetables should be presented in a way that the person they refer to can understand them. Where reading skills are poor a timetable can be created by using pictures that illustrate the activity.

For staff to be able to offer a consistent approach to the clients it is vital that they stick to the activities and timing laid out in the timetable. If variation is allowed, it is inevitable that different members of staff will create different variations, depending on the sort of person they are. Once this happens the point of the timetable is lost. The effort which went into producing it is wasted and the staff team (including you) will be complaining about lack of consistency again.

REMEMBER

Lack of a consistent work practice is inevitably presented as the fault of someone else – when did you last hear someone complaining about their own practice? Until everybody accepts their own personal responsibility for how they behave, admits to making errors, works for improvement and always aims to following the agreed timetable exactly; the clients will not have the reassurance of consistency.

If you identify any changes which need to be made, don't make them yourself; talk to your line manager, ask for time at a staff meeting to discuss and agree the changes.

Always keep IPPs up-to-date AND always keep up-to-date with IPPs.

TASK

Talk to your line manager before starting on this task. Ask him/her to make sure that everyone in the staff team knows what you are working on.

Notes
....

Select an Individual Programme Plan for one of the clients you work with, read it through and make careful notes on its recommendations. Observe the person you have selected and their timetable, for the next five working days. Answer the following questions:

1   In which respects are the plans, objectives and guidelines being effectively followed?

2   In which respects are the plans, objectives and guidelines not being effectively followed?

3   What deviations from the plan did you notice?

4   Does every client have an individual timetable, produced in a way which they can understand, and available to them at all times?

5   If the answer to question 4 is No, why not?

Use Worksheet 23 at the end of the section to write the answers to the questions above and to make recommendations.

AUTISM FOCUS

CONSISTENT WORK PRACTICE